About the Autho

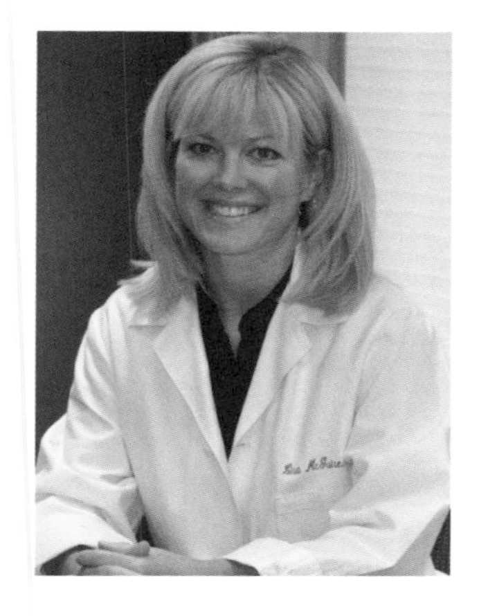

Lisa M. Davis, Ph.D., PA-C, is an obesity expert whose areas of specialty include internal medicine, weight management, and diabetes education. She received her Ph.D. in Nutrition from the Johns Hopkins Bloomberg School of Public Health, where her research focus was examining the role of dopamine in obesity and addictions. Dr. Davis is Vice President of Research and Development at Medifast, Inc., heading the Nutrition Support, Product Development, and Clinical Research divisions. She has been Principal Investigator on several clinical research trials evaluating the safety and efficacy of products and programs. She was previously a faculty member at the Johns Hopkins Bloomberg School of Public Health, and a clinician at the Johns Hopkins Weight Management Center.

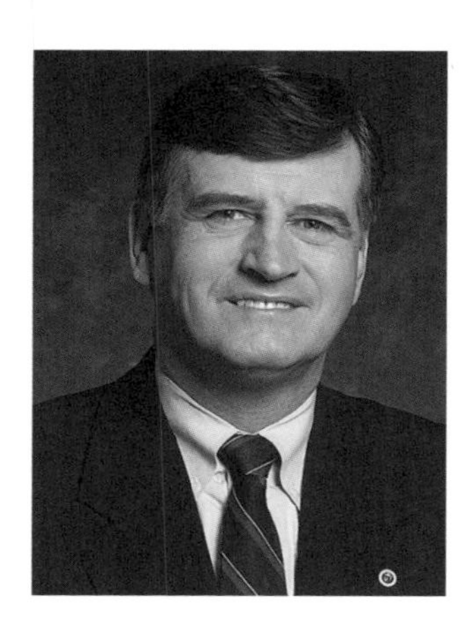

Brad MacDonald is a retired Colonel who served his country as a Marine Corps officer for 26 years. Mr. MacDonald's professional career includes extensive executive experience in the nutrition, weight loss, and health industries with organizations such as Carnation Company, American Brands, Vitamin Specialties, The Marine Corps Exchange System, and Begley Drug Stores. Mr. MacDonald joined Medifast in the late 1990s as CEO and has led the expansion of Medifast's clinically proven line of products to over 70 food items by developing new categories of foods to serve consumers better, maintaining a company commitment to research and development, and expanding the business to multiple channels of distribution to meet the needs of individual consumers. He is committed to proliferating meal replacement technology for weight management and improved health outcomes. Mr. MacDonald's most significant accomplishment in his business career has been establishing a health network which extends the use of Medifast products in a weight-maintenance program as the co-founder of Take Shape For Life, a division of Medifast. He is now the Executive Chairman of the Medifast Board of Directors, focusing on strategic business issues and building relationships in the community. Mr. MacDonald is also a member of the Board of Trustees at Stevenson University (formerly Villa Julie College) in Stevenson, MD.

The Secret Is Out

What physicians have always known about weight loss.

Lisa Davis, Ph.D., PA-C.
and Col. Bradley T. MacDonald, USMCR (Ret)
with a foreword from Dr. Wayne S. Andersen

The Medifast® Program

This book is not intended to take the place of medical advice from a trained medical professional. Readers are advised to consult a physician or other qualified health professional regarding treatment of their medical problems. Neither the publisher nor the author takes any responsibility for any possible consequences from any treatment, action, or application of a medicine, herb, or preparation to any person reading or following the information in this book.

The mention of specific organizations or authorities in this book does not imply endorsement by the publisher. The mention of specific organizations or authorities in this book does not imply their endorsement of this book or the Medifast Program.

Medifast makes no claim that results are representative of all participants on the Medifast Program. Medifast recommends you consult with a physician before starting a weight-loss program.

The Secret Is Out: The Medifast Program
What doctors have always known about weight loss
Lisa Davis, PhD, PA-C and Col. Bradley T. MacDonald, USMCR (Ret) with a foreword from Dr. Wayne S. Andersen

Published by Medifast, Inc.
11445 Cronhill Drive, Owings Mills, Maryland 21117

version 022410_TSIO

Dedication

To my wife Shirley who has been dedicated to Medifast in good times and bad and developed long-term friendships and professional admiration for a special group of tenured Medifast associates who manufacture and provide customer care for thousands of our doctors and customers throughout the United States. Special thanks to Charlotte Stack, Janet Grube-Parks, Nadine Pilker, Beverly McClendon, and Cheryl Smith, who have been loyal and passionate supporters of Medifast. They are the reason that Shirley and I were able to take the risk and re-energize the Medifast brand. They represent the finest tradition in Corporate America of dedicated associates who were willing to sacrifice to make the company work. God Bless them and all hard-working Americans.

- Col. Bradley T. MacDonald, USMCR (Ret)

This book is intended to present what Medifast® believes to be scientifically sound, and recommended, guidelines for the use of our products and programs. So whether you are a medical professional, Health Coach, or person who has just embarked on your own weight-loss journey, please refer to this book as a key resource and educational tool to assist your success while following Medifast.

For medical professionals, *The Secret Is Out* contains medically approved protocols and program materials to help you help your patients achieve and maintain safe and effective weight loss. For Health Coaches, counselors, and individuals looking to lose weight, please use this book is an educational resource and tool. For individuals who are not medically trained or who have purchased this book to lose weight themselves, know that you are receiving a resource that extends beyond these pages with access to Medifast's medically trained staff. Should you need clarification or have questions about anything related to Medifast, Medifast's professional, medical, and customer service staff are available to assist you.

Acknowledgments

Medifast would not be here today if it were not for the genius of William Vitale M.D., the founder of Medifast in the early 80s, and his son Jim and daughter Susan Boone.

Thanks to Lawrence Cheskin M.D., Director of the Johns Hopkins Weight Management Center, who has been an objective scientist and clinical examiner in weight loss and has validated the effectiveness of Medifast products and programs in his research. Without this research, Medifast would not have attained the widespread doctor acceptance and acclaim it has today.

Special thanks to our Food Scientist Ayfer Hoffman for her outstanding product development work. Her efforts have been instrumental in the success of the Medifast Program today.

Today, the vision of establishing a health network of trained professionals who are knowledgeable and proficient in Medifast products and programs is a reality because of the unique partnership of Dr. Wayne Andersen and Leo Williams, III, who lead the Take Shape For Life® division of Medifast, Inc. One of the most exciting accomplishments of my career has been the co-founding of the Take Shape For Life health network using the Medifast Program with Dr. Andersen who is one of the most passionate physicians and health providers in this great nation of ours.

Special thanks to the Augustinian Order of Friars at Villanova University for their outstanding moral, ethical, and academic support, led by Fr. Donald F. Reilly, OSA. The initial study that led to today's successful Medifast business model would not have happened if they had not been willing to lend a hand to a friend who was sinking fast. Their moral leadership yesterday and today on our Board of Directors makes Medifast, Inc. a model of good Corporate governance that has helped us build a special relationship with our employees, vendors, and investors.

Thank you to Robert Barbash who played a critical role with the reconciliation of liabilities during the company's turnaround.

At a time when we could not recruit or afford a professional staff, Stevenson University, formerly Villa Julie College, (located in suburban Baltimore, MD) provided a group of professional interns like Jaime Elwood and Shannon Davis who today are key executives in our organization.

Special gratitude to Rich and Betty Law who took a great risk moving from Texas to Owings Mills, MD, to provide exceptional information systems and nursing support. Nurse Betty made a difference helping Medifast patients get well, along with Dr. Andersen's wife Lori. We have the best medical team in our industry. A special thanks to the Medifast Nutrition Support team—Joni Rampolla, RD, LDN; Jessica Kiel, RD, LDN, CPT; Laura Ford, RD, LDN; and Tammy Hutchisen, RD, LDN, CPT—for their contributions to the Medifast programs in this book.

I want to give special thanks to my daughters: Margaret MacDonald Sheetz, who left a promising legal career to join Medifast at a time when she not only supervised manufacturing and customer service, but also answered the phones and provided customer service because we could not afford an expanded staff; and Kellie MacDonald Pizzico, who left a fast track career at Xerox to join our sales team and lead our clinic operations in Florida.

Finally, I want to thank my brother Mike MacDonald, Director of Medifast and President of Worldwide Marketing at Xerox Corporation, for providing sound counsel and advice in the most treacherous financial time in our company's history. Together with Fr. Joe Calderone OSA, Mike McDevitt, Mary Travis, and Scott Zion, they provided sound strategic advice that helped Medifast become a success story in our industry.

Today, Medifast is one of the fastest growing companies in the weight-loss industry because of the special intelligence and leadership of Michael S. McDevitt, a former Blackstone Group investment banking executive who became our Vice President of Finance, then our President, and is now our CEO. His dedication and insights into developing the Medifast business model are the driving force behind our success in the twenty-first century.

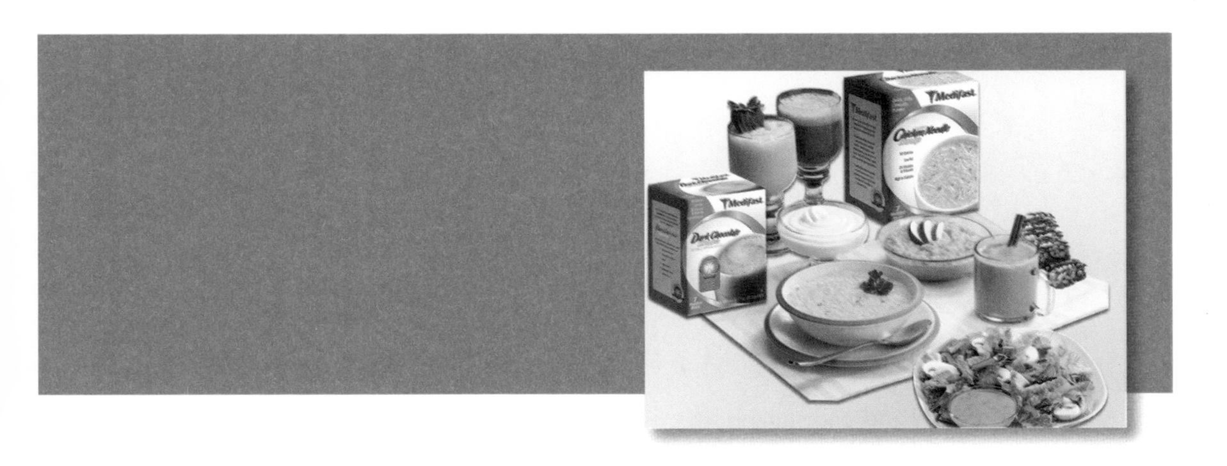

Contents

Foreword	vi
Introduction: What are we up against? Why Medifast?	1
Toni Altamar's success story	6
Chapter 1: Why other diets don't work: Debunking the myths	7
Chapter 2: The doctors' best kept secret: Why Medifast works	15
Thuxoan Tsang's success story	24
Chapter 3: Hunger and your brain	25
Jeff Heck's success story	33
Maureen Heck's success story	34
Chapter 4: Pathways to health: Quelling inflammation and reducing oxidative stress	35
Chapter 5: Personal journey: Getting into the Medifast mindset	49
Debbie Dewey's success story	70
Chapter 6: The Medifast 5 & 1 Plan®	71

Chapter 7: Transition and Maintenance 79

Ted Hasse's success story 100

Chapter 8: Get moving with Medifast 101

Shannon Wollam's success story 112

Chapter 9: Soy and your health: Discovering the truth 113

Tanya Sexton's success story 118

Chapter 10: Medifast for Women's Health 119

Denise Brown's success story 129

Kelly Ellis' success story 130

Chapter 11: Medifast for Men's Health 131

Brent Mouzalkis' success story 140

Chapter 12: Nutritionally enhanced food for health 141

Mary Jane Medlock's success story 158

Chapter 13: Weight-loss medications and obesity surgery 159

Chapter 14: On your way! 173

Ron Taylor's success story 175

Nnedi Uzowihe's success story 176

Chapter 15: Recipes and meal plans 177

References 199

Index 209

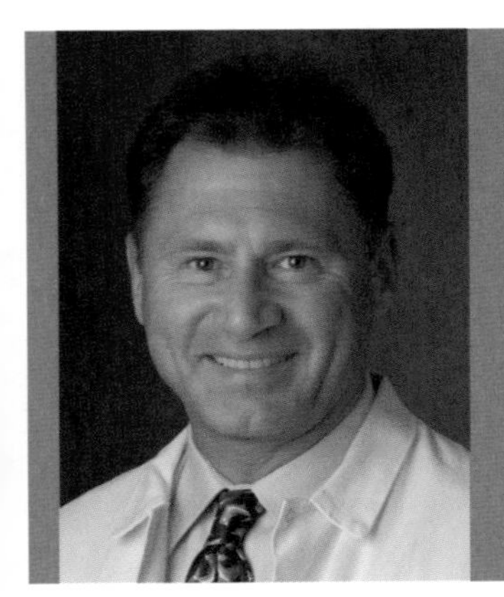

Dr. Wayne S. Andersen is a board certified Anesthesiologist and Critical Care Specialist. He has served as Chairman of the Department of Anesthesiology and Director of Critical Care at prestigious Grandview Hospital. Graduating first in his class from medical school, he helped pioneer the emerging specialty of intensive care medicine. Dr. Andersen's certainty that innovative nutritional intervention is essential in both disease management and creating optimal health has been validated by his experience as the Medical Director of Medifast and co-founder of Take Shape For Life. Chosen as one of the top physicians in nutritional intervention in the country, he is currently working with a team of like-minded medical professionals to provide access to a comprehensive leading edge program, which assures long term solutions to a variety of today's most pressing health challenges.

Foreword

When the absolute necessity of making safe, effective, proven nutritional intervention easy for the individual became clear to me, Medifast was the only logical choice. The company's twenty-five plus year history as a leader in meal replacements, its reputation for excellence backed by clinical studies with Johns Hopkins, NIH, and the real-world experience of more than 20,000 doctors and millions of people, are proof of the truth of their leadership in the field.

One of the exciting parts of Medifast meal replacements is that by providing these safe, great-tasting, easily prepared meals, we can make an immediate change in a person's life. The individual begins feeling great, looking good, and in a very short period of time, is gaining the confidence needed to sustain the critical initial weight-loss phase.

While our patients are enjoying their newfound levels of energy and self-assurance, we teach them the components necessary for lasting, long-term success.

We have over 100,000 people who in the last five years have dramatically altered their health for the better, forever.

From the diabetic mom in Dayton, Ohio, who is now free from the necessity of taking 18 medications and has dropped 10 dress sizes, finally being in control of her health and her life ... to the vascular surgeon in Florida who has lost over 100 pounds and is now a vitally alive example for his patients ... our products and programs are revolutionizing health across America.

I am convinced that our portion-controlled, low-fat meal replacements have the ability to raise the bar, setting a new, higher standard for health and happiness.

Obesity is the logistical and psychological result of our flourishing economy, and conventional solutions are simply not working!

Medifast meal replacements provide a proven power tool to not only furnish a reliable, easy way for people to lose weight safely and quickly, but also provide an excellent means to maintain a healthy lifestyle for the rest of their lives.

We know we should eat smaller meals throughout the day, yet most people struggle with even eating once! Now, the large variety of healthy, easy-to-prepare meal replacements with identical nutritional footprints in a pleasing variety of tastes and textures, allows us to give people a lifeboat of healthy portable nutritious fast foods. No longer do you have to be a hungry victim of dangerous, over-processed fat and sugar-laden nutritional pollution.

Imagine a program that takes the guess work out of calorie counting and food preparation!

In addition to providing the perfect solution to weight management, our Medifast Meals can help people with previously debilitating diseases such as diabetes with a safe, medically proven alternative to help manage their illnesses. I am convinced that sooner than later, we will find that nutritional intervention can even reverse some of these diseases.

I believe that during this decade, our work with our clinical partners will move meal replacements (in tandem with a program of supported lifestyle change) ahead of medications and surgery as the first choice in disease treatment and prevention.

If you could use a program that was safe, proven, and without the side effects of medicines and surgeries to accomplish long-term success—would you do it?

Our goal is to provide the products and program that people can do from the comfort of their own homes and working lives at a cost equivalent to their normal grocery bill. Now that's a program that will actually work!

Please, I encourage you to make the time to read this whole book. It's quick and easy (just like our program itself). It will explain the secret of safely losing weight, which has long been known to the medical community.

Good luck, and know you are taking the first step to an amazing journey of optimal health!

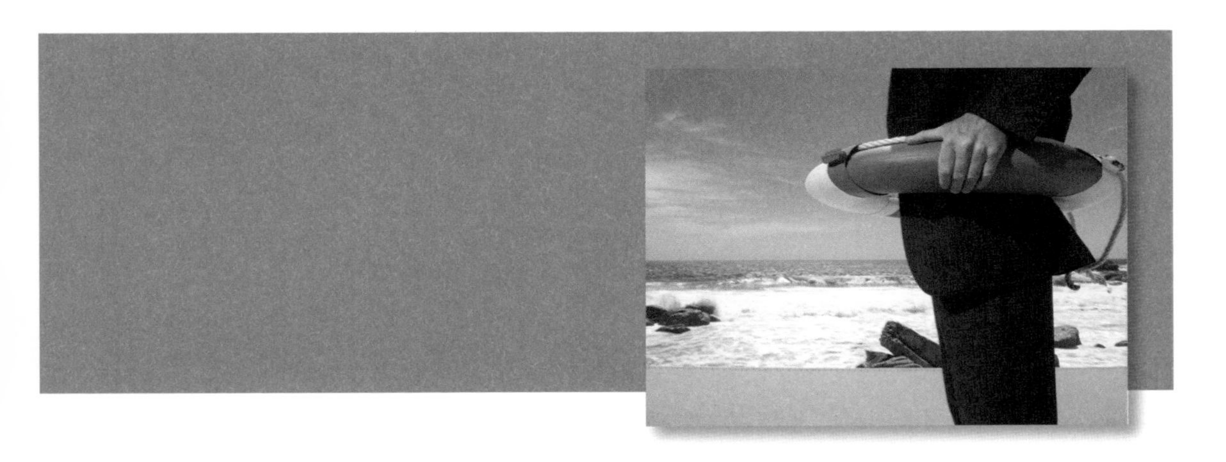

Introduction

What are we up against? Why Medifast?

If you have a copy of this book, you probably bought it with the hope that it will provide the solution to your dieting dilemma—the solution that all other diets have failed to produce for you until now—the key to losing weight and keeping it off, for good.

If you are struggling with a weight problem, you are in good company. The reality is that most of us are already overweight, and it's likely to get worse. Even for those of us who are not currently overweight, there is a very good chance that we will be. The most recent statistics from the Framingham Heart Study show that, even if we are of normal weight at age 50, half of us will become overweight, and one in four of us are doomed to become obese.[1]

The obesity paradox

Everyone knows that being overweight is bad. We know the physical, psychological, and financial tolls that it takes on us as well. We also know that just a ten-pound (or five-percent) weight loss can dramatically improve our physical and psychological health, and often reduce the need for expensive and side-effect-prone medications. Why then, despite constant reminders that obesity is bad and thinness is good, and with access to more dietitians and diet doctors than ever before, are we unable to lose the pounds and keep them off? Why are we condemning ourselves to a host of health problems, a poorer quality of life, and the likelihood of premature death, when all we need to do to prevent this fate is to lose weight?

The struggle with our body weight has not come about because we are uneducated or unmotivated. In fact, most of us are highly educated about nutrition, are motivated to lose weight, and have tried just about everything to drop the extra pounds. We are losing the battle because we are fighting against something that is larger than ourselves. Our genetics may predispose us to a certain degree of thinness or fatness, yet our gene pool has undergone very little change since prehistoric times. Despite our relatively stable genetic make-ups, the sky-rocketing rates of overweight and obesity suggest that environmental factors are more to blame.

While it is true that we as individuals are largely responsible for our own personal environments and behaviors in them, we have essentially no control over the larger environment framed by political, socioeconomic, and commercial forces. These forces have created today's "obesigenic," or fat-promoting, environment. This largely explains why more Americans are overweight compared to any other time in our history.

The public health burden associated with being overweight has ramifications similar to that of tobacco. According to the British Heart Foundation (2004), obesity is associated with a decrease in life expectancy of approximately nine years, mostly due to increases in cardiovascular disease (CVD) and cancers. If that isn't bad enough, some researchers believe that the rising rates of childhood obesity will likely make this new generation the first to have a shorter life expectancy than that of their parents. The sad reality is that our schedules are too busy, and lifestyles too hectic, to be successful at losing weight and keeping it off when we are up against America's fat-promoting environment.

What are we up against?

Politicians and industry leaders have both played roles in making sure that a surplus of unhealthy foods are readily available to us. They are bigger and tastier than ever before, and are more affordable than most healthful foods. Fast foods, convenience foods, and commercially baked goods are inexpensive and taste good because they are loaded with fat and sugar. High-fat, highly sugared foods provide the greatest number of calories for the smallest price. This means that those who can afford less (and ultimately spend less money) paradoxically get more calories and fat. As you might imagine, this affects those in lower- to middle-income brackets the most. Obesity rates in these socioeconomic strata prove it. The problem has gotten so bad that some public health researchers have suggested placing a "twinkie tax" on junk foods. A twinkie tax would theoretically level the playing field between the cost of healthy and unhealthy food items, so that one red pepper would no longer cost more than an entire box of donuts.

Another trick by the food industry designed to keep us coming back for more is the use of high fructose corn syrup (HFCS), found in everything from soda to baked goods. Between 1970 and 1990, the consumption of HFCS increased more than 1,000 percent, far exceeding the changes in intake of any other food or food group.[2] HFCS now represents more than 40 percent of caloric sweeteners added to foods and beverages and is the only sweetener used in non-diet soft drinks in the United States today. It is probably not by chance that the increased use of HFCS in the United States mirrors the rapid increase in overweight and obesity. HFCS does a bad job at signaling the brain to let it know you are full and the end result is that you continue to eat without ever really feeling full.

Another major problem is portion size. Larger portions began in the 1970s and have continued to rise just as levels of overweight and obesity have among Americans. As Greg Critser points out in his provocative book *Fat Land*, the serving-size shift primarily took place in the fast food industry where big chain restaurants (e.g., McDonalds) decided they could get a higher profit margin by serving larger servings of french fries, compared with the profit margin of the standard hamburger. He also points out that fast food vendors accommodate two-income wage earners who were on the run, and likely appreciated the cheap and convenient Happy Meals.[3]

While likely not on purpose, the reality is that America's plump-promoting network of politicians and industry leaders has failed us. The fat-promoting environment, created in the name of free trade, translates into cheaply made, high-fat, highly sugared foods in serving sizes two to four times the standard size. The use of cheap artificial sweeteners like HFCS, and their poorer ability to signal fullness to the brain, allow us to remain hungry and continue to eat. The availability of these fat-promoting foods, plus the fact that they taste good and are cheaper than healthier food items like fresh produce and seafood, are major reasons why Americans are overweight. Our heavy workloads, increased levels of stress, and on-the-go lifestyles make these foods particularly appealing because they are convenient, tasty, and take less time to prepare than most healthy food items. Couple this with decreased levels of physical activity for the average American, and it is clear that today's fat-promoting reality provides a significant barrier to fighting the war against overweight and obesity. Given this toxic, obesigenic environment, what can we as individuals do to tackle the high odds we face?

The doctor's secret

Our fat-promoting environment encourages us to eat more and exercise less. Most people choose to combat this environment by diet-hopping. There is a multi-billion dollar per year industry out there that supports their efforts. Unfortunately, our environment (coupled with our busy schedules and hectic lifestyles) makes it hard to stick with a diet long-term.

There is a way, however, to stop the diet-hopping cycle, protect ourselves against the fat-promoting environment, and follow a healthy eating plan for life that has been scientifically validated in clinical studies. Medifast has been "the doctor's secret" to dieting success since 1980. Originally available only by prescription, Medifast is now directly available to everyone. With Medifast, we can outsmart the slender-sabotaging environment and be victorious in our weight-loss efforts. Medifast has been used and recommended by more than 20,000 doctors since 1980, and is well-respected within the medical profession.

Key reasons why Medifast works:

- In the short term, Medifast breaks the vicious cycle of overeating by providing a simple, easy solution to making meal choices in our busy, stressful lives.
- In the long run, Medifast helps by providing what we know is best: a structured plan that provides six meals per day. Medifast helps us get the number of meals that we need without having to make impractical lifestyle changes.
- Medifast enables us to "step back" from the obesity-promoting environment by allowing us to avoid difficult food situations and vast choices, while learning to structure our eating patterns in a healthier way.
- Medifast is portion-controlled, providing the optimal number of calories for healthful weight control.
- Medifast helps reduce hunger pangs associated with traditional diets. People feel full, and are therefore more apt to stick with the program.

- Medifast is scientifically proven to promote weight loss and improve health outcomes like diabetes and high cholesterol.
- Medifast is tailored to meet individual needs. There are several nutritionally enhanced Medifast Meals to address a range of health concerns, including the Medifast Plus line for: Diabetes, Coronary Health, Joint Health, and Men's and Women's Health.
- Medifast has been carefully crafted to meet the specific needs of both men and women.

As we enter the new millennium, we owe it to ourselves to ask, "What can I do to save myself from becoming yet another statistic in the fight against overweight and obesity?" So many of us have tried and failed with countless diets, but this time will be different. At Medifast, we have considered the fat-promoting environment that we are up against, and have devised a strategy to help successfully overcome it.

The rest of this book is devoted to explaining the Medifast strategy and how to carry it out. The first few chapters provide a more in-depth discussion about how other diets work (or don't work) and what makes Medifast different. The next few chapters detail the Medifast specifics. These chapters begin by providing motivation for adopting the healthy behaviors that will help you succeed with your weight loss efforts, followed by the details of the Medifast 5 & 1 Plan. After that, you will learn about the support systems Medifast provides during both the weight-loss and weight-maintenance phases of your program. Information on exercise basics and suggestions for types of exercise that you can do is also included.

The remainder of this book is designed specifically to show you how Medifast's nutritionally enhanced meals can be used to meet specific health and gender needs. It will even show how Medifast can be used safely with more extreme measures of weight control, like appetite suppressants and after gastric bypass surgery. The book wraps up with an overview of what you've learned, and sets the stage for taking the critical step toward reaching your goals.

Toni Altamar

lost 50 pounds with Medifast

"I was always very thin when I was young. I had four children and put on a little weight, but after the last two, the weight just stayed with me. I still didn't consider myself heavy, but in my late 30s and into my 40s, the pounds seemed to multiply.

"I tried the low-carb trends, but was always hungry. I was scared of taking diet pills and wanted to lose weight in a healthy way. Medifast is perfect, because I'm never hungry, the plan is easy to follow, and there are no health risks for me.

"Within the first week of starting Medifast, I could see results. It was very motivating for me to see a change so quickly; every week was another reason to cheer myself on! Plus, my husband and I had started Medifast together, and we succeeded together. Now we cook at home most evenings and have fish, salad, and a fresh vegetable. We eat mostly from the Lean & Green Meal list.

"My family can't believe my appearance; neither can my co-workers and the lady who's altering all of my old clothes! I'm in sales and travel a lot, meeting new people and entertaining clients. After losing weight, I am doing all of these things with more ease and self-confidence."

Results will vary.

This success story lost weight using a Medifast Weight Control Centers Program.

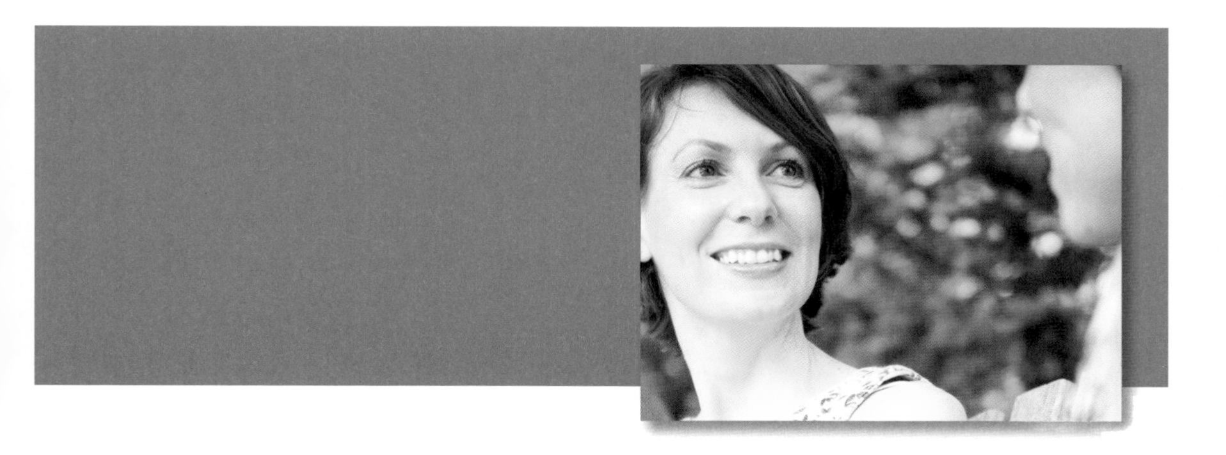

1 Why other diets don't work

Debunking the myths

You should now be familiar with the obesity-promoting environment. To combat it, you've hopped from diet to diet, yet nothing seems to work. The purpose of this chapter is to clear up mistaken beliefs that exist about how all those diets you've tried work (or don't work). In order to do so, there are some myths about dieting that we'll need to debunk.

Myth: You will lose weight if you follow the Food Guide Pyramid Diet.

Reality: The Food Guide Pyramid Diet may help, but it must be portion-controlled.

The USDA's Food Guide Pyramid and Dietary Guidelines recommend a low-fat, higher carbohydrate diet with 20 to 35 percent of your total calories coming from fat, 45 to 65 percent coming from carbohydrates, and the remainder coming from protein. Nutrition experts created the Food Guide Pyramid so that the typical American would know the number of daily servings to eat from each food group as part of a healthy diet.

Serving sizes, however, are often not the same between the Food Guide Pyramid and the nutrition facts food label. To add more confusion to the mix, many Americans think of serving sizes as being larger than they actually are. Let's use a serving of pasta as an example. Many of us think that a plate of pasta equals one serving size. The reality is that one serving size of cooked pasta is equal to one-half cup. That means the typical plate of pasta likely contains three to four one-half cup serving sizes. And that is before we add the garlic bread. Our mistaken beliefs about proper serving sizes allows us to eat far more calories than are actually recommended, and far more calories than we know we are eating.

A 2004 study in obesity research validates this point.[4] Dieters lost more body weight and fat on a portion-controlled diet of prepackaged foods than on a self-selected Food Guide Pyramid diet of the same nutritional makeup (55 percent carbohydrate, 25 percent protein, and 20 percent fat). The bottom line is that precise portion control is an extremely important factor in weight-loss success, and the use of prepackaged entrees is an effective method for achieving this. That is why Medifast's portion-controlled entrees help people successfully lose weight.

Myth: **Cutting carbs is the key to weight loss.**

Reality: **The bottom line is cutting *calories*.**

Whether counting fats, carbs, or points, the bottom line to making all diets work is cutting calories. That is, taking in fewer calories than the body uses. Another way to think about this is that we must burn off more calories than we eat. (What differs among the popular diets out there, like Atkins, South Beach, and Weight Watchers, is picking the popular macronutrient—fat, carbohydrate, protein—of the day to limit in the diet.) In this way, carb-lovers can follow high-carb, low-fat diets, and meat-lovers can follow high-protein, high-fat diets, and we are expected to believe that both can cause weight loss.

Regardless of the type of diet you have been following, there is an underlying myth to these diets: There is nothing special about minimizing fats or carbs that causes you to lose more weight. The truth is that weight loss on any diet does not occur because you have limited (or eliminated) a specific macronutrient (fat or carbs). It occurs because by limiting the consumption of that macronutrient, you are ultimately decreasing your total intake of calories. In other words, the fundamental principle behind the success of any weight-loss plan is no more complicated than the picture below.

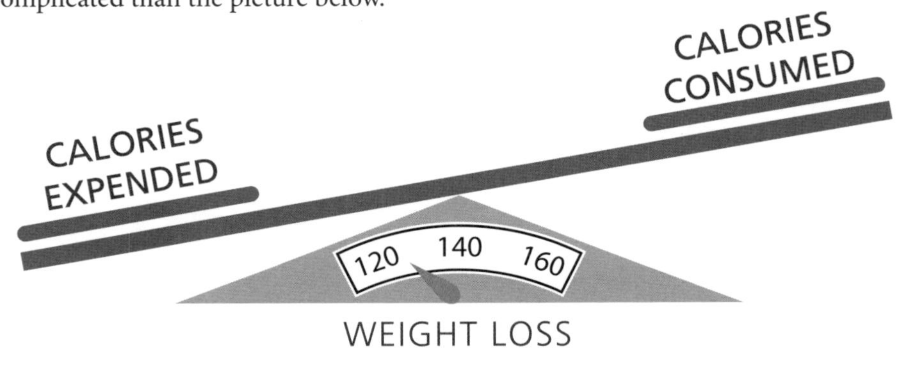

Let's use the Atkins diet as an example. The Atkins diet claims you can eat as much protein (and fat) as you want, as long as you restrict your intake of carbohydrates to practically nothing. For many people, eating just protein (and no carbs) is difficult. So, people often end up eating less food than they would normally eat, and end up losing weight because they are taking in fewer total calories.

The scientific evidence backs this basic dietary principle. After reviewing more than 100 diet studies, researchers found that weight loss from low-carb diets comes from eating fewer calories, not from eating fewer carbs or any other magic nutritional combination. Studies show that the best predictors of weight loss appear to be caloric intake and diet duration, the longer the better. This means that there is nothing special about limiting carbohydrate intake, in particular, that causes weight loss independent of calorie reduction itself.

While total calories is really what counts when it comes to weight loss, there are some differences among the macronutrients themselves that everyone should know. The first is that all macronutrients have a unique number of calories per gram.

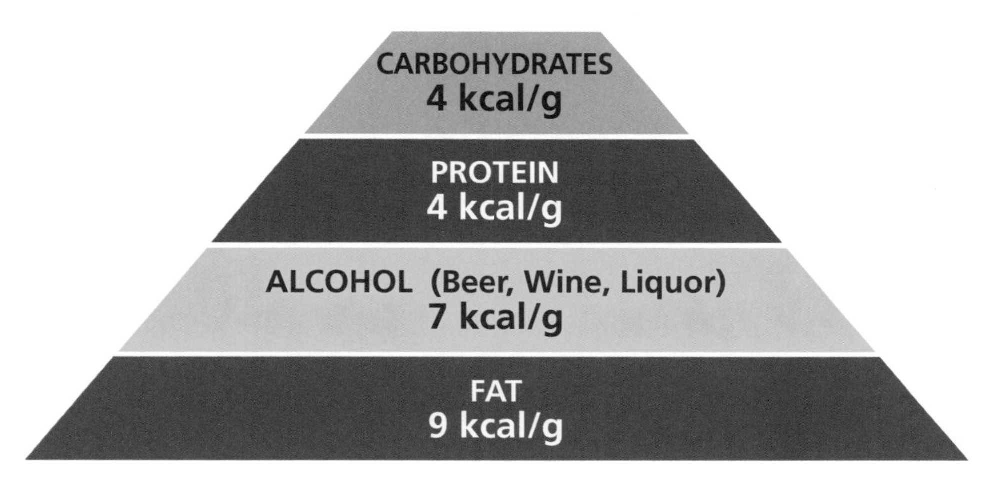

Figure 1. Macronutrient density hierarchy

Looking at this macronutrient hierarchy, you can see why limiting your intake of fat (and alcohol) makes sense when you are trying to lose weight. It also shows the flawed logic of diets that allow an unlimited amount of fat, like Atkins does.

There are 4 main reasons why eating fat makes us fat:

1. Fat has more than twice the number of calories (for the same weight of food) than carbohydrates or protein.

2. Fat promotes overeating by making the flavor and texture of foods more appealing.
3. Fat is less filling than protein and carbohydrates, so we eat more of it before we feel full.
4. When we eat too many calories, carbs get burned first (before fat and protein), and fat gets stored.

All of these reasons support low-fat diets when it comes to losing weight. Understand, however, that the reason for the weight loss on a low fat diet is not because you are restricting the fat itself, it is because by restricting your fat intake, you are decreasing your total intake of calories.

> ***REMEMBER:*** There are good fats and bad fats. Your diet should be low in saturated fats (butter, lard, Crisco) and trans fats (hydrogenated and partially hydrogenated oils), and higher in monounsaturated (olive and canola oils) and polyunsaturated fats of the omega-3 series (fatty fish, like salmon). Lower amounts of saturated fats, and higher amounts of monounsaturated fats and polyunsaturated omega-3 fatty acids, have been shown to have a positive effect on your cardiovascular health. Furthermore, a certain amount of fat is necessary for essential bodily functions and the absorption of fat-soluble vitamins.

Myth: High-fat, low-carbohydrate diets are healthy.

Reality: NOT TRUE!!

The aim of high-fat, low-carbohydrate diets is to force the body to use fat as its main energy source. Basically, you cut out virtually all carbs from your diet and increase your intake of protein and fat. You can't eat pasta, bread, rice, or fruit, yet you can eat unlimited amounts of meat, cheese, and butter. That's why the Atkins diet seems so wonderful. It's a bacon lover's dream.

The Atkins diet claims that by switching to a diet that's extremely low in carbohydrates, insulin production is decreased, food cravings are dampened, and stored fat is burned off. So, you can eat steak, eggs, cheese, and butter, but virtually no bread, pasta, fruit, or sugar—even many vegetables are banned. What they fail to tell you is that the same argument could be applied to high-fiber complex carbohydrates as well. High-fiber complex carbs swell in your belly and take up space, thereby minimizing food cravings. They also slow down the speed that sugar is released into the bloodstream, decreasing insulin requirements.

In addition, many low-carbohydrate diets, (like Atkins) are high in fat, saturated fat, and cholesterol. Unlimited amounts of fat (especially saturated and trans fats) increase various health risks. While probably less harmful in the short term, numerous medical associations have warned that over time, high-fat diets can lead to heart, kidney, and liver problems. Another concern about high-fat, low-carb diets is a deficiency of essential vitamins and nutrients that can occur if supplements are not taken. High-fat, low-carbohydrate diets are low in several nutrients: vitamins A, B6, D, and E; thiamin; folate; magnesium; iron; zinc; potassium; and fiber. You can only get many essential nutrients from fruits, vegetables, and grains. Low-carb diets only allow very small amounts of fruits and vegetables—well below the amounts needed to deliver your recommended daily allowance. The bottom line is that these diets lack the nutrients essential for good health.

Finally, high-fat, low-carb diets are also likely to encourage yo-yo dieting, (vicious cycles of losing and regaining weight) which has been shown to be a health risk. We've all done it. Like a yo-yo, the numbers on the scale go down, but then almost as quickly those numbers go right back up. It's frustrating, self-defeating, and with each attempt, the hope of ever being successful and healthy seems farther and farther away. Additionally, the studies on yo-yo dieting have shown some concerning consequences:

- It may increase the amount of fat in the body relative to lean tissue.
- It may redistribute fat sites. For instance, fat which was lost from the hips and thighs may be regained in the abdomen. (Excess amounts of fat in the abdomen may increase the risk of cardiovascular disease.)
- Diet cycling may also increase the risk of high blood pressure and heart disease.
- Repeated dieting and regaining may impair the body's weight-regulation system. It seems the more diets we go on, the harder it becomes to lose weight.

Myth: We must learn *how* to eat right to keep the weight off permanently.

Reality: In reality, learning *how* to eat right is just not enough.

Many good diets rightfully advise that in order to keep the weight off, you must learn *how* to eat right. There is no argument there—just inadequate advice because the *how* that is being recommended is precisely the problem. The *how* is just not realistic given today's time-limited, stressful lifestyles. It is a challenge to find the time to gather all the necessary ingredients to make multiple healthy, portion-controlled meals a day, and quite frankly, access to fast food is just too easy. The combination of no time and easy access to unhealthy foods packaged in large serving sizes is a recipe for disaster. In addition to the major time commitment, having to make lots of day-to-day food choices and keeping track of points or grams is difficult for many. The *how* is why traditional diets fail and at least 75 percent of dieters regain the weight. It's why, despite being better-educated about the harmful effects of being overweight (and having access to more nutrition-trained healthcare providers), more Americans are overweight or obese than are normal healthy weight. Many of us know how to lose the weight and still cannot. We can't because knowing how to lose weight is simply not enough.

The *how* of many diets simply tells us that we are personally responsible for changing our habits and environments to make them conducive to weight loss. But, the *how* doesn't consider the larger forces, the fat-promoting environment described in the introduction, over which most of us have little or no control. Knowing *how* might be enough if we all lived in ideal situations. Surely, if we were all independently wealthy, had our own personal chefs, and junk food was simply not available at convenience stores and fast-food chains, we could all be thin. The bottom line is that just knowing *how* to lose weight is not enough. Knowing *how* simply does not offer strategies for helping to combat the fat-promoting environment and for sticking to diets in today's world. Medifast is a successful plan because it is as much a strategy and lifestyle as it is a diet.

Myth: I can't lose weight because I am a junk food junkie.

Reality: This may be true—but it's not entirely your fault—and you can change!

Even if you have an addictive personality when it comes to food, there are other influences out there making your food cravings and choices seem out of control. Knowing what these influences are, so that you can plan for them instead of react to them, will put you in a position of greater control.

Let's begin with manufacturers who know that we have an inherent desire for the taste of yummy foods. Big industry sugar pushers know that sweetened, high-fat foods are essentially addicting to genetically vulnerable types, and use it to their advantage to keep us coming back for more. The reason why we are addicted to these foods and tend to binge on them is because they can act like drugs in our body, stimulating the brain to release certain "feel-good" chemicals, known as neurotransmitters. Opioids and dopamine are two of these feel-good chemicals that are released in response to eating (or even smelling) sweetened foods.

Just as some of us are more predisposed than others to alcohol, drug, or smoking addictions, some of us are more predisposed than others to food addictions. Those of us who have addictive personalities respond strongly to the release of these neurotransmitters to achieve temporary feel good feelings. Unfortunately, the feel good feelings don't last very long, and are often followed by irritability, mood swings, and fatigue. Our temporary "high" followed by bad feelings like irritability and fatigue that make us want to feel good again. So we go back for more of what we know made us feel good before. It is easy to see how a vicious cycle can develop. For more information about this topic, see chapter three.

The food industry is in tune with this phenomenon. They are also keenly aware that the way they manufacture their foods make them provocative to those susceptible to addictive eating behaviors. Yet, in order to continue manufacturing junk food without having to be accountable, they argue personal responsibility. Food manufacturers use the personal responsibility argument when it comes to eating junk food the way tobacco companies do when it comes to smoking cigarettes. That way, food manufacturers can keep store shelves stocked with junk food and the tobacco companies of the world can keep dolling out cigarettes.

In order to make up for our junk food weakness and binge-eating activities, we look for quick and easy solutions to break the cycle and reverse the damage. The easy solutions we look to are fad diets that promise quick results, like the Atkins diet. The problem with these quick-fix diets is that they foster cycles of yo-yo dieting, which ultimately ruins our physical and psychological health, as well as our weight-loss efforts over the long term.

The reason for identifying industry forces that we have little or no control over is not to totally remove personal responsibility from the equation. The reason is to make you aware of the market forces out there so that you can thoughtfully prepare for them, as opposed to just mindlessly reacting to them. If you are prepared, you are much more likely to make wiser food choices.

By avoiding junk food and making wiser food choices, you can actually train your taste buds to prefer the healthy ones. Retraining your taste buds to prefer healthy foods over junk foods can and does take place over time. Some of you may already be familiar with this concept, like when you switched from regular to diet soda or from whole to skim milk. Now, you probably say you can't stand regular soda or whole milk, which you used to love. The point is, we don't have to be slaves to our taste buds. We can send our taste buds to "healthy foods bootcamp" so they can learn to shun the old, unhealthy favorites.

Why other diets fail

Many popular diets fail because they fail to recognize and offer effective solutions for tackling the challenges over which we have little or no control—challenges of the fat-promoting environment. Other diets, (even good ones) fail because they do not provide a tool or strategy that helps prevent relapse in the face of the powerful draw of junk foods themselves. That is what sets Medifast apart from the rest. Medifast allows us to escape from the clutches of our obesity-promoting environment by providing structure and better eating patterns in the context of a nutritionally enhanced, satisfying, and filling diet. View Medifast as a strategic tool of defense against an environment that is working against our weight-loss efforts. Medifast is not just a diet, it is a tool to help you achieve a healthier lifestyle.

2 The doctors' best kept secret

Why Medifast works

Before we reveal to you why Medifast is the doctor's best kept secret to losing weight and keeping it off, let's clear up any misconceptions you may have about diets that use pre-packaged, portion-controlled, nutritionally enhanced meals. These types of diets are not just liquid diets. They are not a quick fix solution that leads to yo-yo dieting. People do not pile the weight back on once they return to normal eating habits. In fact, all of the known scientific evidence points to just the opposite, that dieters lose weight and improve their health, provided they receive advice and stick to eating a healthy, balanced diet once they transition off the program. The results of randomized controlled trials published in the medical literature show that diets based on the same principles as Medifast are effective in reducing everything from body weight to blood sugar levels to high cholesterol levels. Given this degree of scientific validation, it is of no surprise that Medifast has been clinically proven to work, and over 20,000 doctors have recommended Medifast to their patients.

The concept behind Medifast

Pre-packaged, portion-controlled, nutritionally enhanced meals may not have been a concept necessary in the 1950s, but these meals are essential for many in the new millennium. Whether ideal or not, the reality is that many of us simply do not have the time to prepare multiple healthy meals and snacks everyday. In the absence of having healthy, portion-controlled foods prepared for us, we end up making poor food-related decisions. For many of us this occurs because we wait until we become ravenous to eat, then are bombarded with too many readily available, unhealthy food choices in today's fat-promoting environment. It's a lot faster and takes less effort to grab a milkshake and fries after working all day, running errands, and spending any meaningful time with your family than it does to prepare and cook a healthy meal.

Incorporating healthy, portion-controlled entrees as part of a healthy diet can aid in breaking that cycle of impulsive food buying based on environmental food cues. Since the benefits of Medifast Meals are that they are convenient, portion-controlled, and keep us feeling full, we won't give in to temptations based on the sight, smell, or convenience of foods. Because you eat every two to three hours, you will have fewer hunger pangs, so you won't feel the same desire to binge on sweet, high-fat foods.

The basic fundamental by which Medifast Meals work is by substituting a fixed portion of food that is made up of less energy (calories) than the food usually eaten at a given meal. The energy difference between the Medifast Meal and the usual meal is what leads to weight loss or weight maintenance. Portion-controlled entrees that are designed to replace the foods usually eaten at meals (particularly when combined with behavior-modification techniques) have the best track record among the dozens of weight control strategies scientists have tested. That's why portion-controlled Medifast Meals can be viewed as your strategic tool to dieting success, even when other programs have failed you.

Medifast—A scientifically proven diet plan

Stop counting calories, carbs, or points, and let Medifast do it for you. Medifast's pre-measured meals are low-calorie, low-fat, nutritionally balanced, portion-controlled meals designed to replace the ones we would have normally consumed—the ones that made us overweight in the first place.

Research at a major university teaching hospital and the National Institutes of Health (NIH) shows that Medifast Meals are very effective and safe for both short- and long-term weight control. The research conducted by these renowned institutions adds to the mounds of existing scientific evidence showing that pre-packaged, portion-controlled meals produce significantly better results than traditional diets. They outshine other diets when it comes to short-term weight loss, long-term weight maintenance, and improvements in health like diabetes and high cholesterol. Let's take a closer look at the research.

Weight loss

Major research study

For more than eight years, the Johns Hopkins Weight Management Center in Baltimore, Maryland, has used Medifast products for its very low-calorie weight-loss programs. In clinical studies, researchers found that the vast majority of patients (91 percent of males and 72 percent of females) lost more than 40 pounds on the Medifast Program in 16 weeks. Researchers concluded that weight loss programs by Medifast provide a safe, effective means of weight reduction and are accompanied by significant improvements in systolic and diastolic blood pressure readings, total cholesterol, and triglycerides.

National Institutes of Health (NIH) obesity research study

Twenty-four obese women who entered a medically supervised weight loss program followed a 1,200 kcal/day American Heart Association step-2 diet, with or without the use of Medifast supplements. Over a 13-month period, the women on Medifast lost, on average, 15 pounds of body weight, 10 pounds of body fat, and lowered both their cholesterol and glucose levels.

Diabetes

The efficacy of Medifast Plus for Diabetics was also clinically studied by comparing it to basic nutrition recommendations provided by the American Diabetes Association (ADA). Results of the study show that individuals with type 2 diabetes, using Medifast Plus for Diabetics, lost twice as much weight after 34 weeks as those following the ADA's recommended food guidelines and were twice as likely to stick with the diet.

Why Medifast works

So now that we know Medifast works, let's get into the specifics about why Medifast Meals work in the short term to get the weight off, and help to maintain weight loss in the long run. There are at least six reasons why Medifast works:

- Is portion-controlled
- Provides five structured meals/day
- Helps you stick with the diet
- Minimizes food choices

- Is satiating (keeps you feeling full)
- Breaks the cycle of bad habits/food addictions

Medifast meals are portion-controlled

With marketplace portions now two to four times the size of standard serving sizes, and because calorie content increases with portion size, portion-controlled meals are an effective way to reduce total calorie intake and body weight.

Portion-controlled meals are also helpful in preventing the over-consumption of food. The tendency to passively overeat foods has been shown in children. Doubling the serving size of a lunch entrée led to a 25 percent increase in the amount of calories consumed during the lunch meal, and a 15 percent increase in total caloric intake for the day. Yet when children were allowed to serve themselves, they chose smaller portions and consumed 25 percent less of the entrée than when they had been served a large entrée portion.

Medifast provides five to six structured meals per day

Structured diet plans consisting of five to six portion-controlled meals each day are associated with better outcomes in terms of weight loss, weight maintenance, and improvements in blood sugar and cholesterol levels. The same benefits are not found, however, when the five to six meals consist of super-sized portions of high-fat, high-sugar convenience foods at the expense of fruit, vegetables, dairy products, and whole grains—a result that often occurs when we are on-the-run. Chaotic eating patterns that result from our busy lifestyles also make it difficult to judge exactly how much food we have consumed, which can lead to overeating.

Eating six healthy meals a day takes planning and effort. Since most of us do not have the time to plan and make six meals each day, Medifast helps by providing portion-controlled cuisine that is easy to prepare and healthy. Having to eat six times a day staves off hunger and decreases your risk of over-consuming unhealthy, fat-promoting foods. What's more, Medifast Meals are fortified with the essential vitamins and minerals that many people are missing from their high-fat, high-sugar diets.

Medifast helps you stick to the diet

One of the reasons portion-controlled, pre-prepared meals successfully aid weight loss is because dieters don't have to prepare meals. Traditional diets require that you weigh and measure foods, choose between food options, and monitor your portions. Medifast provides a convenient, portion-controlled, no-brainer approach to weight loss, so you can stick to it. That's why research has demonstrated that twice the number of dieters were able to stick to their Medifast weight-loss plans compared to dieters on a traditional diet. Better compliance with the diet equals better results.

Medifast minimizes food choices

While variety may be the spice of life, when it comes to losing weight and keeping it off, having a greater variety of food choices may actually sabotage your dieting efforts. According to the latest research from the National Weight Loss Registry, minimizing food choices may help to curb your appetite.[5] It turns out that men and women who were most successful at maintaining a weight loss of 30 or more pounds for at least one year were the ones who ate a diet consisting of a limited variety of foods.

The weight-loss benefits of limiting the range of foods one eats may also be related to a phenomenon called "sensory specific satiety." The way sensory specific satiety works is that the more you eat of a specific food, the less satisfaction you get with each bite, so your desire to continue eating that food fades. Since your desire to eat that food fades, you eat less overall. But, be careful not to take a bite of a different kind of food, because that will stimulate your desire to continue eating.

Medifast is satiating (keeps you feeling full)

You can stay full on Medifast because you get to eat your meals more frequently. It's hard to be hungry when you eat six times each day. Also, Medifast Meals are high in protein (soy protein) and fiber, both of which keep you feeling fuller, longer. So that you can see the difference between types of food in terms of the satiety (or fullness) they provide, and why Medifast chose to create low-fat, high-protein, high-fiber meals, we have created a 7-tiered hierarchy of satiety (see figure 1). The order of satiation (or fullness) goes from the top

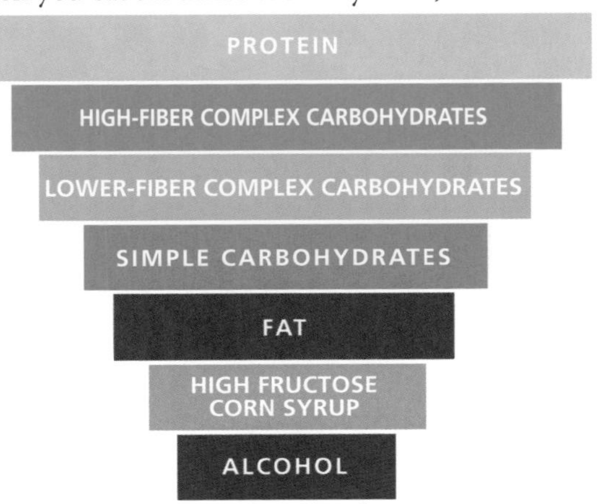

Figure 1. 7-tiered hierarchy of satiety

of the hierarchy with protein as most filling, to the bottom of the hierarchy with alcohol as least filling.

Protein (of all kinds) is the most filling type of food, followed by high-fiber complex carbohydrates (e.g., fruits, vegetables, legumes, whole-grain breads), then lower-fiber complex carbohydrates (e.g., pasta, potato without the skin, white bread), simple carbohydrates (e.g., table sugar, candy, marshmallows—the sweetness in snack and fast foods), fat (e.g., butter, oil, avocado), high fructose corn syrup (found mostly in soda and baked goods), and alcohol (which includes wine, beer, and spirits). Let's take a closer look at some of the differences.

Protein

Scientific evidence strongly indicates that protein is the most filling nutrient. There are different kinds of protein, such as egg albumin, wheat gluten, and soy (to name a few). Medifast chooses to use soy protein for its satiating effects, as well as for its beneficial effects on health. Studies show that the satiety values of different protein sources vary little, making soy a wise choice for both satiety and health reasons.

> With Medifast Shakes, you have the choice of two different amounts of protein. Individuals who want more protein may use Medifast 70 Shakes (14 g protein/meal). For individuals who need, or prefer, a slightly lower protein diet, Medifast 55 Shakes (11 g protein/meal) may be more appropriate.

High-fiber complex carbohydrates

Medifast Meals are rich in fiber. In addition to five pre-measured Medifast Meals per day, you eat one "Lean & Green" Meal every day. This meal will also be filling because it consists of a protein source of your choice plus a salad or vegetable (high-fiber complex carbohydrates). The high-fiber, high-water content of low-fat, carbohydrate-rich foods, can enhance the feeling of fullness both during and between meals.

Carbohydrates vs. Protein

Referring back to the macronutrient density hierarchy from chapter 1, you can see that there is essentially no difference in between the number of calories per gram of carbohydrate and per gram of protein. There are some differences between the two macronutrients, however, that are worthy of mention.

- It takes a little more energy for the body to metabolize, or break down, a protein than it does a carbohydrate, so you may burn a few more calories by eating protein-based foods than carbohydrate-based foods.

- Protein ranks higher on the hierarchy of satiety than carbohydrates, and protein is particularly more satiating than simple carbohydrates like sugar.

While you may burn slightly more calories with protein than carbs, and protein may be more filling, you may actually get fewer calories from carbohydrates than you do from protein. Let's see how.

When we assign a number of calories to a macronutrient, we do so based on dry weight as opposed to wet (cooked) weight. The dry weight of a carbohydrate equals four calories per gram; however, when it gets diluted by water and fiber, the average energy content decreases to one-and-a- half calories per gram. For example, by boiling your pasta in water on the stove, you reduce its number of calories per gram from four to one-and-a-half.

The take home message is this: In the overall analysis, there is probably very little difference between the energy content of protein and high-fiber complex carbohydrates. In the long run, a healthy diet should include them both.

Carbohydrates vs. Fats

A similar energy density comparison may be made between complex carbs and fats. The difference in energy density (number of calories per unit volume) between carbs and fats helps explain why carbohydrates are more filling. The difference between fats and carbs is actually even greater than it appears. That's because the volume does not change, when you take a dry fat and cook it. The volume doesn't change because fat is not made up of fiber and does not soak up water. Carbs, on the other hand, are made up of fiber and do soak up water. As result of this dilution, cooked (or wet) carbs have a larger volume than do dry carbs, but fewer calories per unit volume. In other words, you get more calories for the same amount of dry carb than you do for cooked carb. We said pasta has about four calories per gram when dry in the box before cooking. A typical serving size is two ounces dry. Once it is cooked, it may swell with water to several times its dry volume, obtaining an energy density per unit volume lower than the pre-cooked volume. Since cooked (or wet) pasta has one to two calories per gram, you can eat more volume and get fewer calories.

Also, fibrous carbohydrates and vegetables (e.g., lettuce, asparagus, cucumber, broccoli) have very low calorie densities because our bodies cannot absorb the caloric content of fiber. Any food that has a lot of fat in it will have a high-calorie density. Foods that are 100 percent fat have the highest energy density, or the most calories per volume. Consider some examples: olive oil (which is pure fat) contains 1,920 calories per cup, peanut butter has 1,600 calories per cup, and cashews have 780 calories per cup.

High-fructose corn syrup (HFCS)

Finally, HFCS assumes a position close to the bottom of the 7-tiered hierarchy of satiety. The reality is that it contributes very little in the way of satiety, and may not be filling at all since it does not appear to send satiety signals to the brain. The rise in obesity reflects the prevalence of HFCS. Despite the widespread use of HFCS by the food industry (and ironically by the diet industry,) Medifast avoids the use of this sweetener in its products.

The plan that breaks the cycle of bad habits and food addiction

Because you get to eat more frequently, and because Medifast keeps you feeling full, it may prevent you from relapsing into bad eating behaviors. Because you will feel full, you will be less likely to give in to those old triggers that make us want to eat. View Medifast Meals as strategic tools for preventing relapses in an environment full of tantalizing foods. Willpower alone cannot match the prevailing market forces that promote unhealthful foods, making them available for our consumption on every street corner, the way that liquor stores do with alcohol.

How is Medifast different from the rest?

You may be asking yourself what makes Medifast different from other diets that use pre-prepared, portion-controlled meals as a strategy for weight loss? Since many of you are familiar with SlimFast® as a diet plan that incorporates pre-prepared, portion-controlled meals, let's use it as a comparison.

While Medifast and SlimFast® share the same basic fundamental approach to weight loss in that they both provide a structured, portion- and calorie-controlled diet plan, there are at least four important ways Medifast differs from SlimFast®:

- Medifast Meals generally contain fewer calories per serving than SlimFast®. The difference may not seem like much at first, but over time, the seemingly small difference in calories can really add up.
- Medifast avoids the use of high fructose corn syrup. HFCS is found in many SlimFast® meals. This is paradoxical for a diet product, since we

know it does little in the way of signalling the brain that the body is full. HFCS may even trigger excessive consumption of foods.

- Most Medifast Meals are made from soy protein, whereas SlimFast® is made from mostly whey protein. Medifast offers a few whey protein based food choices for the small population of people who may have a soy allergy. Medifast prefers soy protein because soy has a number of important health benefits that whey protein doesn't provide:

  Soy comes complete with all essential amino acids in exactly the right balance to meet your body's needs.

  Soy is a rich source of nutrients, including calcium, iron, zinc, phosphorus, magnesium, B-vitamins, omega-3 fatty acids, and fiber.

  Soy protects against some of the most harmful diseases we face,

  including cancer and heart disease. In recognizing the heart-protective effects of soy, the U.S. Food and Drug Administration (FDA) authorized the use of the following health claim: Consuming 25 grams of soy protein daily, as part of a diet low in saturated fat and cholesterol, may reduce the risk of heart disease.

- Certain Medifast Meals are nutritionally enhanced to meet specific health and gender needs. SlimFast® does not provide products similar to Medifast Plus for Diabetics, Coronary Health, Joint Health, and Women's Health. The problem with promoting the same product to everyone is that we are not all the same. Medifast's unique line of condition- and gender-specific food products effectively solves this problem.

Now that you see why the Medifast Program is right for you, the next chapter of this book will motivate you and get you mentally prepared to begin your Medifast journey toward weight loss and better health. We'll teach you tactics that will help you identify and deal with food cues and diet saboteurs, so that you are in a position of control. You'll learn mindful eating practices that will help you get the most out of your meals.

Thuxoan Tsang

lost 65 pounds with Medifast

"When I got married 14 years ago, I was a size-10 bride and I want to turn back the clock. Well, after 4 children it was time to start taking care of me! I wanted to run, climb, and go crazy with my children.

"My husband and I researched the Medifast Program and philosophy. He liked the fact that the 5 & 1 Plan did not deprive me of carbohydrates, proteins, fats, and nutritional supplements, just calories. We both liked the fact that it was a simple diet, emphasizing drinking lots of water (good for you), finishing the Meals every two to three hours, and having a light meal. Well, that was simple enough; it was time to go for it!

"I opened my first packet, Dutch Chocolate Shake, and was on my way. Each week, I lost 2-4 pounds! I found that it was a no-brainer to follow the diet. I had more time to my day, because I didn't have to worry about eating. I know what I had to eat at what time.

"My husband is so excited about Medifast that he is recommending it to his patients. Since his philosophy remains that he treats his patients like he would treat his wife, he feels that Medifast is currently the state of the art diet."

Results will vary.

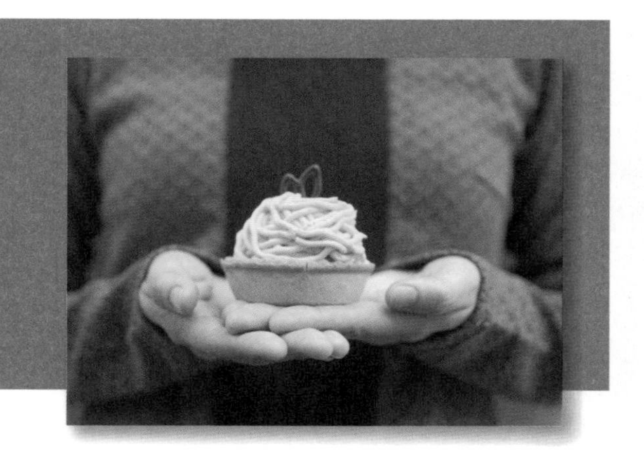

3 Hunger and your brain

Did you ever wonder why so many times after so many meals, you still feel vaguely hungry? Do you long for seconds while your thin friends say they are completely stuffed? Do you love eating foods that other people say are "too sweet" or "too rich?" Maybe at times you've wondered if you were wired differently than these other people. And maybe, just maybe, you weren't so far off in your thinking.

Although for years overeating has been criticized as a lack of willpower, weakness, or even a sin (gluttony, anyone?), science now understands that there can be a physical cause for excessive eating. Under certain conditions, the brain isn't able to understand that you've had enough food and shut off your hunger when it's time to put down the fork. It's very difficult to stop eating when your body is telling you that you're still hungry. Understanding how this process works can help you quit beating yourself up for gaining too much weight—while at the same time, helping you take steps to heal yourself and reverse these trends where you can.

The brain, appetite, and eating behaviors are all incredibly complex, much more so than it's practical to cover here. However, this chapter will give you some insight into your relationship with food by explaining a bit about how your appetite works, what happens when it's not functioning properly, and how you can potentially find the solution to eating more normally.

Food as a reward

When it comes to food, are you one of those folks who would describe yourself as being "driven to eat" or "never satisfied?" Some people tend to have an inborn condition called "reward deficiency syndrome," a problem with the brain's pleasure mechanisms, which are essential to feeling like we've had enough to eat. Individuals with this trait (estimated to be about 30 percent of the general population) seem to have been born with fewer "pleasure receptors" in their brains. These receptors are signaled by "pleasure molecules" to let our brains know when we're content and satisfied. So for people born with a shortage of pleasure receptors, eating an ice cream cone might not be as pleasurable as it would be for someone without a reward deficit.

But having a muted pleasure response to ice cream and other yummy, rich foods does not make people want them less. Rather than saying no to the ice cream, they eat more of it in an attempt to get the pleasurable feeling of eating something that tastes good.

To fully appreciate the concept of reward deficiency, a little bit of background in "Neurochemistry 101" is helpful. Our brains, feelings, and emotions are steered by chemicals called neurotransmitters, and these are made up of molecules. Dopamine is an example, and is known as the "pleasure molecule." This "feel-good" neurotransmitter gets released in response to rewarding activities, including "natural" rewards (e.g., love, reproduction, eating) and "unnatural" rewards (e.g., compulsive overeating, drug use, gambling).[6]

In order for the dopamine to work and be felt by the body, its molecules have to attach themselves to dopamine (pleasure) receptors located in various places around your brain. When pleasure receptors don't work like they should, the reward signal is diminished, driving people to get a "fix" of something in order to feel good. For obese individuals, the fix may come in the form of overeating. Dopamine has been shown to be the primary controller of hunger and the motivation to eat[7] and is also involved in the "rush" (reward value) of food, drink, sex, and drugs of abuse. [8-11]

People prone to obesity may have a tendency to overeat, especially sweetened, high-fat foods, in an attempt to stimulate their short supply of pleasure receptors. However, when they attempt to stimulate these blunted dopamine receptors by overeating to compensate for the reward deficit,[12] they simply desensitize the few receptors they have, and make bad eating behaviors even worse. Figure 1 shows the vicious circle involving low dopamine receptor concentrations, unhealthy eating behaviors, and obesity.

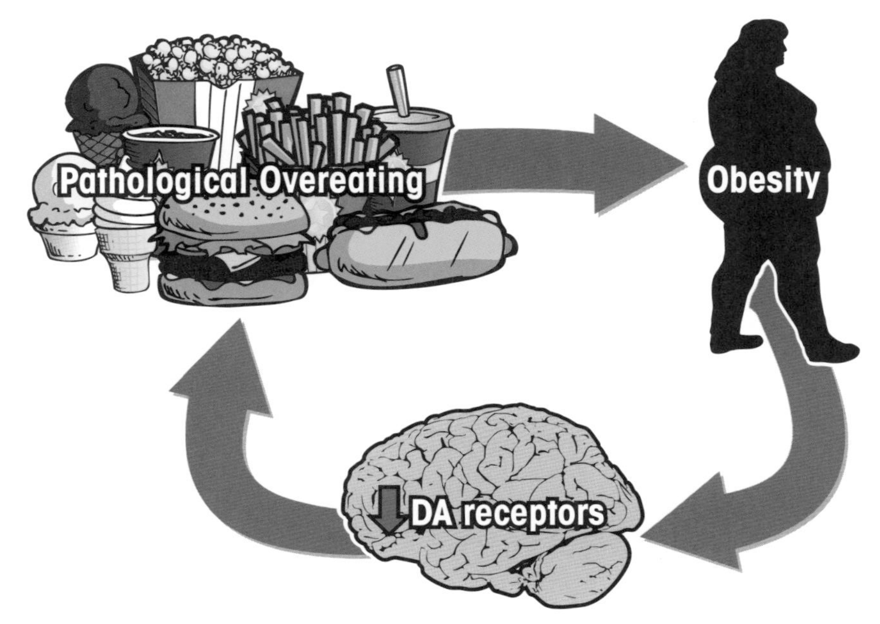

Figure 1. Cycle depicting dopamine (DA) receptor deficiency, overeating, and obesity.

Genetic evidence

Now that we understand the basics of how our brains and our eating give us pleasure, let's switch to another topic that relates to the process: genetics. (Having fun yet?)

Some people with reward deficiency syndromes have a different kind of dopamine receptor due to a specific piece of genetic code called the "Taq 1 A1 allele." According to genetic studies, these people are more likely to be obese[13] or to have substance abuse disorders like cocaine,[14] alcohol,[15] or opioid abuse.[16] This suggests that obese individuals with this piece of genetic code may be prone to abusing food in a way similar to how an addict or alcoholic abuses drugs and/or alcohol. And, if genetics set the stage for overeating, our obesity-encouraging environment adds even more risk with plenty of cheap food that's packed with sugar and calories. Over-consumption of these energy-dense foods leads to obesity.

When looking at where the Taq 1 A1 allele is likely to appear among the general population, we see some patterns. Only 25 percent to 30 percent of the general population shows the variation, but about half of obese people do.[17-18]

The allele shows up in 74 percent of those individuals suffering from both obesity and a substance abuse problem.[19] These trends suggest that for some, overeating may be a kind of addiction with food acting as the "substance of choice." Those addicted to illicit drugs can avoid them; however, no one can avoid food and survive.

So, what's the impact of the Taq 1 A1 allele on the pleasure centers inside your brain? Figure 2 shows you why individuals with the Taq 1 A1 allele experience less pleasure than those with the A2 (normal) allele. The sensation of pleasure begins when dopamine is released from one part of the brain cell, crosses what's called a synapse, and binds to dopamine receptors on the membrane on the other side. If you look at the brain cells of those with the A1 versus those with the A2 allele, you'll see why those with the Taq 1 A1 allele experience less pleasure than those with the A2 allele—there are fewer sites where the dopamine molecules can take hold.

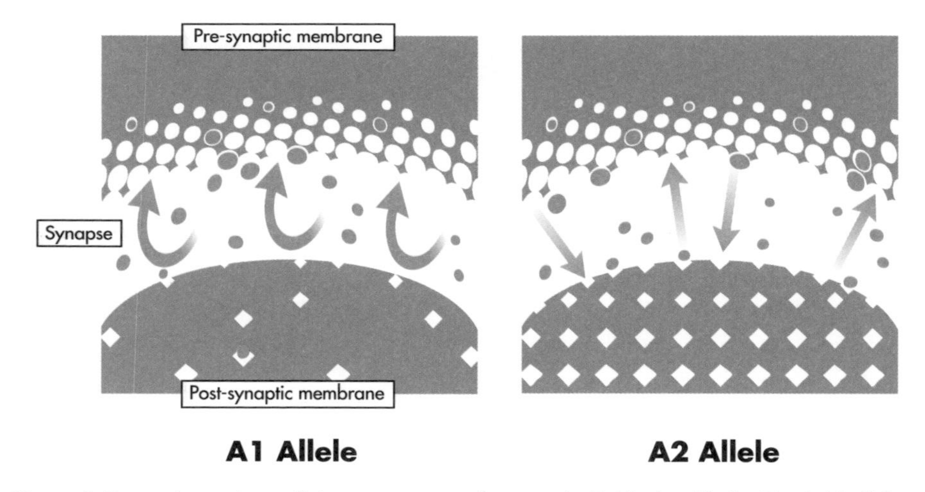

Figure 2. Fewer dopamine or "pleasure receptors" among individuals with the Taq 1 A1 allele.

For people with fewer pleasure receptor sites on their brain cells, adding more pleasure molecules likely won't fix the problem, and in fact, may make it worse. Too much dopamine may overwhelm the receptors and actually prevent them from recognizing the dopamine, causing even less binding. The effect can be disastrous: Many addicts report that they keep "using" in search of that great pleasure they experienced the first time. They continue to ramp up the amount of their substance of choice, requiring more and more each time to achieve the same "feel-good" sensations, until one day, there are none left.

One picture is worth a thousand words

Brain scans show that there are fewer dopamine receptors in the brains of people with the Taq 1 A1 allele.[6, 19-20] Also, obese animals and humans show fewer dopamine receptors in these same regions of the brain than those who are lean.[21-22] In one groundbreaking study,[22] the number of dopamine receptors was shown to be significantly lower in 10 extremely obese men and women compared with 10 lean controls. (See Figure 3.) The study also found that the subjects with the lowest dopamine receptors had the highest body mass indexes.

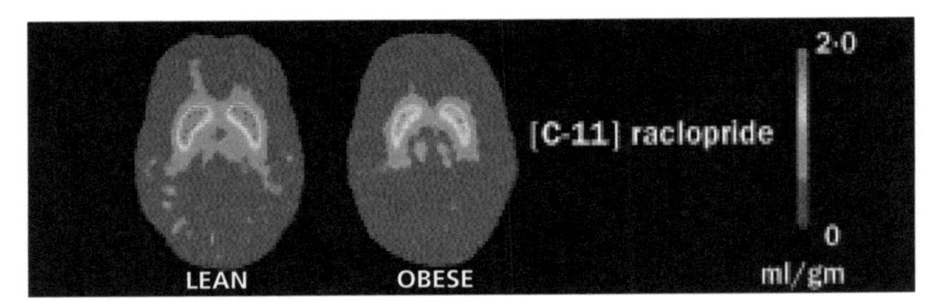

Figure 3. PET scan shows lower dopamine receptors in reward center of obese brain. Images are scaled with respect to the maximum value obtained from the controls and most receptors values represented by the rainbow scale. Red represents the highest value (2.0) and dark violet represents the lowest value (0 ml/Gm).[23]

While the brain scans show a lower number of dopamine receptors in the pleasure center of obese humans in this study, they do not show whether the decrease came about before the obesity (a genetic shortage) or because of it (exhausting the dopamine receptors through overeating calorie-rich, sugary foods). Obesity specialists are still wondering which came first, the chicken or the egg?

A likely explanation is some combination of the two, as is summed up quite nicely by a quote from Dr. Judith Stern, Professor of Nutrition and Internal Medicine at the University of California at Davis: "Genetics loads the gun, but environment [full of easily obtainable high-calorie foods and lacking access to physical activity] pulls the trigger." This situation then leads to the destructive cycle shown in Figure 1.

The picture of addiction and compulsive behavior is incredibly complex and includes not only genetic and neurochemical explanations, but social, cultural, and emotional factors as well. Regardless of what leads to reward deficiency as it relates to drugs, food, or other behavior, the impact on human life is all too well known. As a result of repeating the self-destructive behavior day after day, the person's life becomes more and more chaotic and difficult to manage. Minor consequences, health problems, and other issues are followed by a cascade of more and more serious ones.

Whereas at one point the affected person might not even be aware of a problem, the insidious progression of compulsive eating, gambling, or drugging eventually leads him or her into a lifestyle that's far off the track from where he or she wants to be. Slowly, denial gives way to attempts to stop the behavior and its harsh (even life-threatening) penalties. The unhappy person may reach out for help, but finds that the compulsion to feel even a normal degree of satisfaction or comfort undermines his or her efforts. It takes a lot of courage and hard work to stop overloading the brain's pleasure center, break the cycle, and heal the brain's ability to feel good. Yet when this happens, hope, health, and healing are all possible.

Retraining your brain

Of course, you can't change your genetics or remove the glut of obesity-causing foods in our world. But there are plenty of things you CAN change—especially the foods you choose to eat. Selecting your foods wisely can help instill control back into your life. The following section will provide information on how to "retrain your brain" and take back control of your health.

The last section explained why certain individuals overeat from a neurochemical standpoint. This section explains how you can counteract the discomfort of "reward deficiency" using the Medifast Program. Eating food that gives you a satisfying feeling of fullness can go a long way in helping you feel more comfortable as you make changes to your diet and your life. And eating nutritious, filling foods can also affect other pathways to the brain that interact with the reward center.

Certain foods—primarily those high in sugar and fat—stimulate the release of dopamine in a dose-dependent way, which means the more of these foods you eat, the more dopamine gets released. Eating more for more satisfaction works to a point, but after that, there appears to be a threshold where pleasure receptors get blunted and no longer recognize the signal. If you already have fewer receptors to start with, and now you're blunting the few you have by overeating high-calorie foods day after day, you can see how hard it might be to achieve the feeling of reward over time. Fewer messages get through, and you don't feel satisfaction. Your brain still thinks you're hungry, so you keep eating.

In order to retrain your brain, you should include different types and amounts of foods in your diet This involves switching from high-sugar, high-fat foods to low-glycemic, low-fat foods. Instead of eating large amounts at once, switch to eating five to six portion-controlled mini-meals per day. Small portions of low-sugar, low-fat foods don't stimulate the release of large amounts of dopamine that desensitize receptors, and actually help them regain their sensitivity so you can feel pleasure in eating once again.

Neural firing in the brain is finely tuned to gastric distention and blood sugar levels. The optimal diet provides satiety and blood sugar stabilization while giving pleasure receptors a break so healing re-sensitization can occur. Medifast is a great solution for this task, with portion-controlled, low-glycemic foods that are high in protein and fiber, and offer the highest Fullness Index™ of the top weight-loss plan meals. Medifast Meals are scientifically formulated with just the right balance of ingredients to help you feel full while you eat fewer calories. The bottom line is that you'll get greater satisfaction (satiety) from eating less. Satiety is essential to any weight-loss plan to prevent the discomfort and gnawing hunger that makes you "cheat." When you feel full, you can make smart choices, and soon you will find you are in control of what you eat!

Why Medifast has a high Fullness Index™:

- Protein is the most satiating macronutrient (according to clinical studies as discussed in Chapter 2).
- Excellent source of protein (>10 grams per serving).
- Excellent source of fiber (in most cases, ≥5 grams per serving).

The addition of protein or fiber to a food product will have a positive impact on lowering its glycemic index (how fast it moves its sugars into your bloodstream) and has the effect of making you feel fuller longer. Use the Fullness Index™ calculator below to estimate how filling a food is. Or calculate for yourself how satiating a food is by adding the amount of fiber grams and protein grams, multiplying by 100, and dividing by the number of calories per serving. Let's plug in the values for a Medifast Cappuccino as an example:

Protein	+	Fiber	x	Calories	/	Fullness Index™	=	**18**
14		4		100		100		

There is a common misconception that foods containing lots of fat and calories are the most filling. Let's use the Fullness Index™ calculator to dispel that myth.

As it turns out, if you consumed a McDonald's® Extra Value Meal® every meal of every day for one week, you would consume on average 2,323 calories, 80 grams of protein, and 19 grams of fiber. Despite all of these calories, you still wouldn't feel very full, since the Fullness Index™ of each meal is only 3.5. In contrast, consider a week's worth of Medifast Meals, which provides more protein and fiber than the McDonald's food, but less than half the calories, and a Fullness Index™ that's four times greater than the McDonald's diet.

Many diet plans and products claim that they are filling. A head-to-head comparison of daily meals shows that among the most popular diet plans, Medifast is the most filling, outperforming the others by nearly two to one in terms of Fullness Index™.

Weight-loss plan	Daily calories	Daily protein	Daily fiber	Fullness Index™
NutriSystem®	1,195	75	24.5	9
Weight Watchers®	1,312 (24 points)	72	25	8
Jenny Craig®	1,315	66	14.5	7
Medifast®	**962**	**115**	**27**	**14**

Values are averages based on one week's worth of food on different diets. The higher the Fullness Index™, the more satiety you get with each calorie. Calories, protein, fiber, and Fullness Index™ data are the summary of research performed by Associate Director GPPS at Penn Medicine, Jacqueline McLaughlin, between June 1, 2008 and December 31, 2008.

From your first taste of your first Medifast Meal to your final weeks in Maintenance, you'll feel fuller, more comfortable, and more in control. You will stop giving in to reward deficiency behaviors. And that's how Medifast helps you lose weight and break the cycle of overeating—for good.

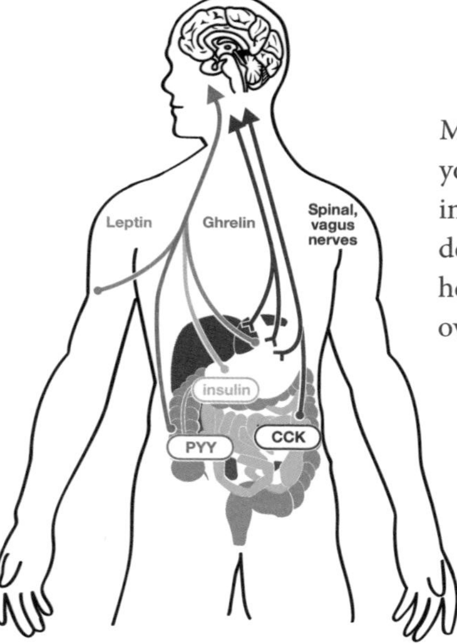

Figure 1. Satiety messengers signaling the brain that the stomach is full (or to stop eating).

Jeff Heck

lost 94 pounds with Medifast

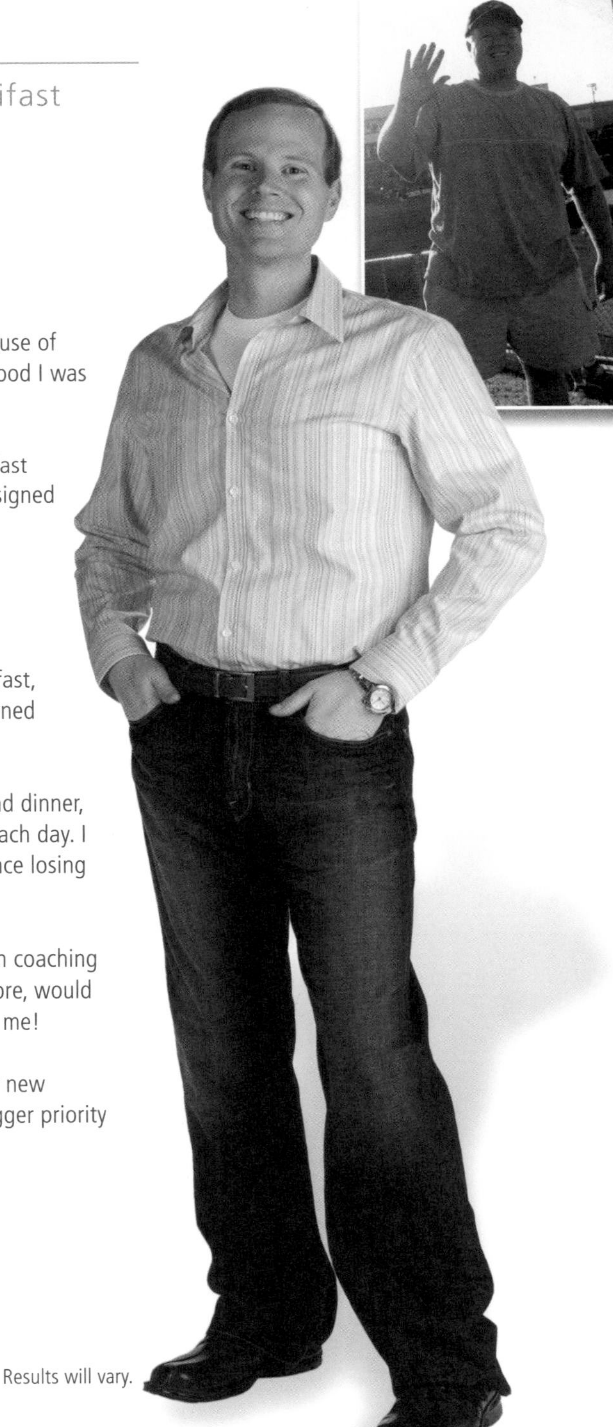

"I was always athletic as a kid, but because of high-fat, home-cooked meals and junk food I was also always overweight.

"When my wife decided to try the Medifast Program, I wanted to support her and I signed on too.

"Medifast was great during a busy workday, as well as business travel.

"Not only did I lose 94 pounds on Medifast, going from a 44 waist to a 32, but I learned how to eat to sustain my weight loss.

"I used to only eat twice a day, lunch and dinner, but now I eat 6 small, balanced meals each day. I have gained amazing self-confidence since losing weight with Medifast.

"I am much more outgoing and I'm even coaching my son's Little League team, which, before, would have been too much in the spotlight for me!

"My wife and I are so excited about our new lifestyle; we are making date-night a bigger priority now!"

Results will vary.

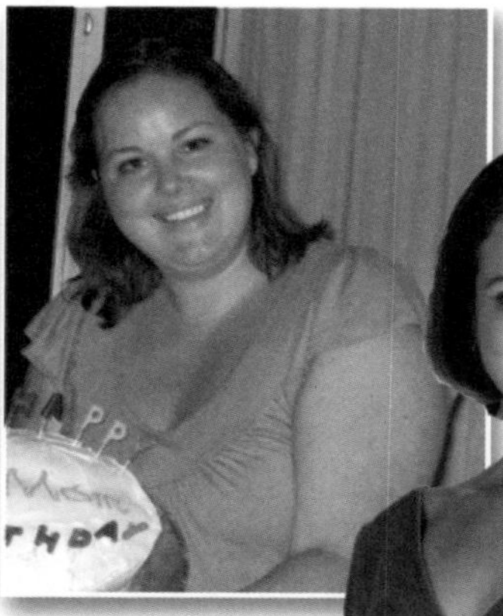

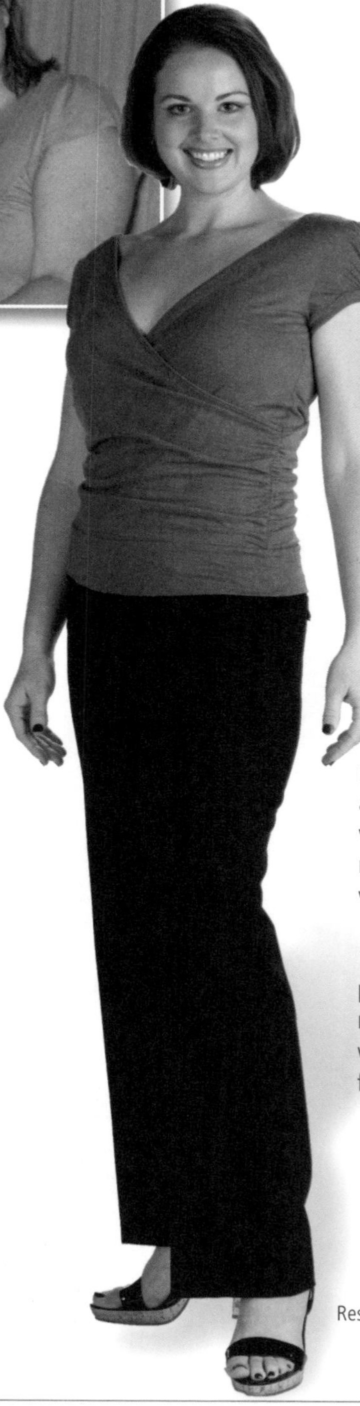

Maureen Heck

lost 75 pounds with Medifast

"I was always on the chubby side growing up and have struggled with my weight pretty much all my life, but I didn't get really heavy until I got married.

"Finally I realized that I wanted to resolve this issue once and for all before my 30th birthday! I tried to do it with diet and exercise but would always lose motivation and by my 29th birthday I was bigger than ever. I accepted the fact that whether I am 'skinny' or 'fat,' I have a weight problem and will always have to manage what I eat. I did my research and chose the Medifast Program.

"The 5 & 1 Plan took the stress out of dieting: no planning, shopping for, or cooking several meals a day... and no counting! And I still got to eat dinner with my family each night. It was great for a busy mom on the go. The weight came off consistently which kept me motivated to stay on track.

"While on the 5 & 1 Plan I learned to eat smaller portions 6 times a day, and with the Medifast maintenance plan I am confident I will keep the weight off for good! I once wore a size 20, and now fit into a size 8!!"

Results will vary.

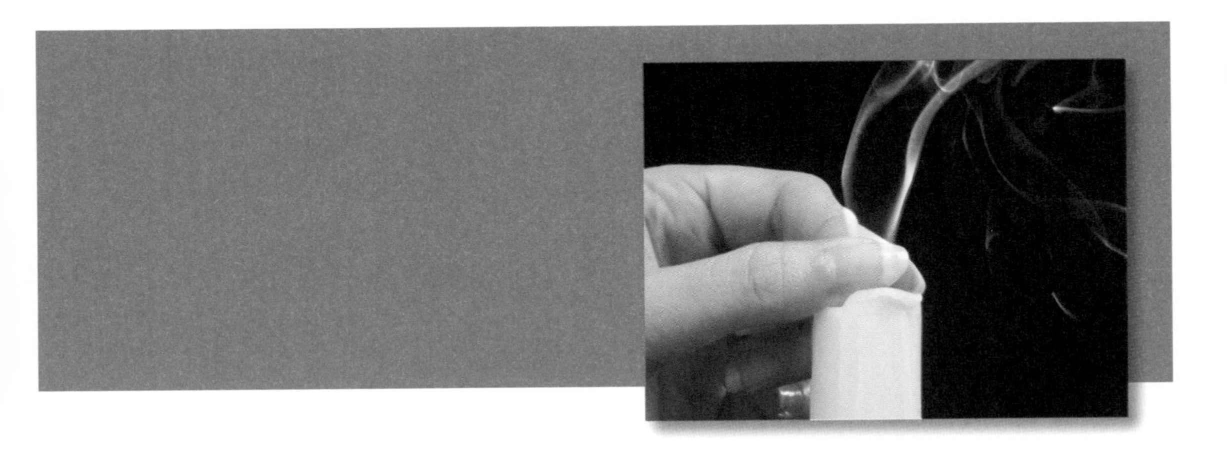

4 Pathways to health

Quelling inflammation and reducing oxidative stress

Inflammation and disease

Many illnesses are caused by specific agents such as bacteria or viruses, but many others are caused by overall health conditions that are preventable, in part through healthy eating. For instance, health professionals are becoming more and more aware that inflammation underlies many of our most common diseases, even the process of aging.

We can all recognize the symptoms of local inflammation: redness, swelling, pain, and heat—think of a fingertip you've just accidentally hit with a hammer, an arthritic knee, or a cut that gets infected. A small, temporary area of inflammation usually doesn't do much harm, but a chronic inflammatory state throughout the body is associated with some serious consequences, including two of the most common killers: cardiovascular disease and cancer.

Obesity shows us a relationship between inflammation and disease. Carrying extra pounds, particularly around the internal organs in the abdomen, is a risk factor for inflammation. This "visceral fat" is metabolically active tissue because it releases a variety of inflammatory molecules into our bloodstream, where they target the cells of all body organ systems, from the lungs to the joints to the central nervous system. Inflammatory molecules may contribute to cardiovascular disease, high cholesterol, asthma, diabetes, rheumatoid arthritis, or and cancer. Inflammation can even affect our mood, aggravating mood disorders, or mental illness.

Health conditions associated with inflammation

System affected	Health conditions
Cardiovascular	High cholesterol or triglycerides, high blood pressure, stroke
Endocrine	Type 2 diabetes, metabolic syndrome, nonalcoholic fatty liver disease
Pulmonary	Asthma
Gastrointestinal	Inflammatory bowel disease (ulcerative colitis, Crohn's disease)
Immune	Rheumatoid arthritis, multiple sclerosis, allergies, psoriasis, atopic dermatitis
Cellular	Cancer (especially breast, colon, prostate)
Psychological	Mood disorders such as major depression, schizophrenia

(Adapted from Rowe, B & Davis, L, 2008.)

Inflammation harms the body by causing too much oxidative stress, which in turn leads to the formation of free radicals that change your body's cells in harmful ways and contribute to disease. Consuming too many calories in the form of dietary fat (especially saturated, trans, and omega-6 fats) and, too much sugar increases the risk for inflammation and oxidative stress in your body (depicted in Figure 1).

Your doctor can give you a blood test to measure inflammation in your body and give you an idea of whether or not you're at risk. The test is for C-reactive protein, which is one of a number of chemical markers in your body that increase in response to inflammation. C-reactive protein levels will show up at high levels in response to an acute injury. But persistent, low-grade levels

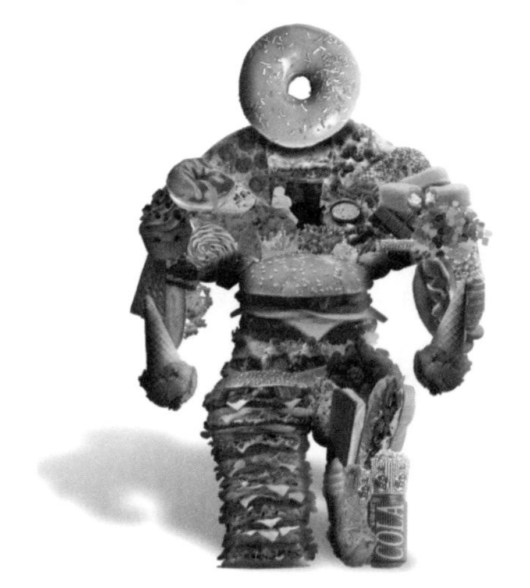

Figure 1. Development of inflammation and oxidative stress

of C-reactive protein are a more worrisome sign that inflammation is setting the stage for chronic diseases like cardiovascular disease and diabetes.

The role of diet in inflammation

When it comes to chronic inflammation, the modern American diet is a definite risk factor. Despite our country's wealth and medical knowledge, the American food industry is not a friend to our cells—or our prospects for a long and healthy life. Whereas in centuries past, Americans lived mostly on lean meat and unprocessed fruits and vegetables, today we gorge on processed foods high in dietary fats and more highly sugared carbohydrates—two of the main nutrients that contribute to inflammatory processes in the body. Some of the most common items on our table are the worst offenders, including sugar-sweetened soft drinks, white flour, processed meats, and foods with unhealthy fats. No wonder more and more Americans are looking closely at the health benefits associated with the so-called "Mediterranean diet," which emphasizes fresh fruits, vegetables, olive oil, red wine, and lean meats, and is associated with decreased inflammation.

Fats in our diet

All dietary fats are not created equal. Not so long ago, all fats were lumped into the "bad" category. The truth is that fats are an essential part of our diet and many fats are actually good for us. Table 2 shows you some different types of dietary fats and how they measure up in terms of health and disease risk.

Table 2. Good and bad fats

Type of fat	Main dietary source	Risk of disease
Monounsaturated	Olive oil, canola oil, peanut oil, almonds, avocados	⇩
Polyunsaturated	Vegetable oils *(corn, soybean, safflower, cottonseed)*, fish	⇩
Saturated	Whole milk, red meat, butter, cheese, coconut oil	⇧
Trans	Partially hydrogenated vegetable oils, most margarines, vegetable shortenings, baked goods, commercially prepared French fries and onion rings	⇧

The good fats

Polyunsaturated fats (PUFAs)

The name sounds like some sort of exotic marshmallow, but PUFAs are fats, and there are two main types of them: omega-3s and omega-6s, with the omega-6s having higher levels of inflammatory potential. Both are essential fatty acids (EFAs), so the body does not make them, and we must get them through the foods we eat. That gives us some control over how much inflammation we introduce into our body through this dietary source.

The past century and its food manufacturing practices have seen an increase in the more inflammatory PUFAs. Before modern processing methods, the ratio of omega-6 to omega-3 fatty acids in the average American diet was approximately 4:1. Today, the same ratio is approximately 20:1.

How do the omega-6 fatty acids cause harm? It's a matter of throwing things off balance at the cellular level. Each cell in our body has a cell membrane that is composed in part of fatty acids—both the omega-3 and omega-6 types. Fatty acids from your diet are readily incorporated into cell membranes, so when it comes to fats, you literally are what you eat: Consuming too much omega-6 and not enough omega-3 can change the cells' membranes and render the cells more susceptible to inflammation.

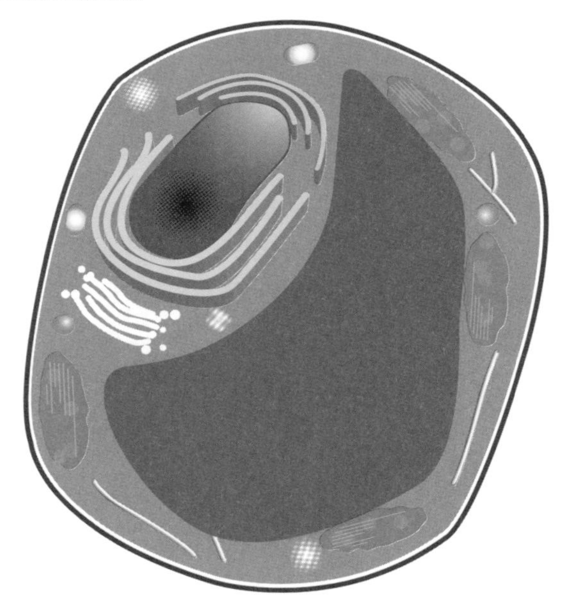

Figure 2: Cell membrane

The good news is that you can balance the ratio of PUFAs by eating more omega-3s and fewer omega-6s. Anti-inflammatory omega-3s will compete for space in the cell membrane and crowd out inflammatory factors.

Recommendations

Currently there is no set recommended daily allowance (RDA) for the intake of omega-3 fatty acids. Many experts agree that omega-3 intake should be between one and two grams per day, and that the omega-6 intake should be no more than four or five times the omega-3 intake. In fact, if you have documented heart disease or high triglyceride levels, the American Heart Association recommends that you eat fish (particularly fatty fish) at least twice per week, and consume two grams of omega-3 fatty acids (with one gram from EPA and one gram from DHA) daily as well.

To decrease the amount of omega-6 fatty acids in your diet, avoid margarine and the following oils: corn, cottonseed, safflower, and sunflower. To increase the amount of omega-3 fatty acids in your diet, incorporate some of the richest dietary sources that are listed in the table below.

Table 3: Dietary sources of omega-3 fatty acids

Food item	Omega-3 fatty acid content (grams)
Fish/seafood *(4 oz)*	
Mackerel	2.2
Sardines	1.8
Salmon	1.7
Swordfish	1.7
Herring	1.4
Scallops	0.5
Tuna *(canned in water)*	0.3
Lobster	0.1
Flax seeds *(1 oz)*	1.8
Tofu *(1 oz)*	0.4
Greens *(½ cup cooked)*	
Spinach	0.1
Kale	0.1
Collard greens	0.1
Oils *(1 Tbsp)*	
Flaxseed	6.9
Walnut	1.4
Canola	1.3
Olive	0.1

Essential1: Heart Health

Even if you are getting some omega-3s through your dietary choices, adding an omega-3 supplement may be a good idea. It's important to understand, however, that not all omega-3 fatty acid supplements are created equal. There are many fish oil supplements on the market, and plenty that don't deliver what you need from them.

The most important thing you will want to pay attention to is how much EPA and DHA an omega-3 supplement contains. The body cannot make use of the parent omega-3 compound (alpha-linolenic acid) as well as it can use EPA and DHA, so you want the highest concentration of EPA and DHA you can find.

Medifast's pharmaceutical grade Essential1: Heart Health Super Omega-3 has the following important qualities:

- A high concentration—and the optimal balance—of ingredients EPA and DHA: Two softgels contain 720 mg EPA and 480 mg DHA.
- The optimal 1.5 EPA:DHA ratio for cardiovascular health.
- Purified deep sea fish oil from clean seas.
- Molecular distillation to ensure the absence of impurities, including PCBs, mercury, and other contaminants.
- Third-party testing to guarantee nutritional content and purity.

How omega-3 fatty acids enhance your overall health

Omega-3s are associated with improvement in cardiovascular risk factors through decreasing:

- Risk of arrhythmias, which can lead to sudden cardiac death
- Triglyceride levels
- Growth rate of atherosclerotic plaque
- Blood pressure (slightly)

Omega-3s support the body's natural anti-inflammatory response, and can reduce joint pain and swelling.

Omega-3s may help with mental disorders and emotional disturbances such as depression and anxiety.

Omega-3s enhance the body's anti-inflammatory response.

Omega-3s promote a healthy immune system.

Omega-3s may decrease cancer risk (particularly breast, colon, and prostate cancer) according to several studies.

How omega-3s optimize weight control

Together with moderate exercise, omega-3 supplements can reduce body fat mass.[24]

Omega-3 supplements can reduce body fat mass in people with diabetes.[25]

Organic flaxseed oil. Flaxseed oil is a good source of the two essential fatty acids that are required for the structure of cell membranes, and, because they are unsaturated, they help keep those membranes flexible. Ingredients in flaxseed oil also help maintain the nervous system and calm inflammatory reactions. Flaxseed oil also contains compounds that act as antioxidants.

Allergy concerns. Fish allergies are caused by fish proteins, which are filtered out of fish oil when it's extracted. Still, some contamination of the oil with small molecules of such protein is possible, so those with a fish allergy should discuss the use of Medifast's Essential1: Heart Health Super Omega-3 supplement with their physician. A fish oil supplement should be safe for use by those with a shellfish allergy since the process doesn't involve the allergens that cause shellfish allergy.

Monounsaturated fats (MUFAs)

Monounsaturated fats (MUFAs) are "good" fats, and are associated with lower levels of inflammation. MUFAs are found in high concentrations in olive, canola, and peanut oils. Monounsaturated fats have a proven benefit in heart disease and cholesterol reduction. Olive oil, in particular, may have unique additional anti-inflammatory powers because of its antioxidant components such as carotenoids and flavonoids (natural substances that provide the good-for-you color that occurs in vegetables and fruits). Newly pressed extra virgin olive oil (the most flavorful kind, and with the most antioxidant benefit), also contains oleic acid, a substance that has similar anti-inflammatory potency to nonsteroidal anti-inflammatory drugs.

Bad fats

Saturated fats

Saturated fats have had an unsavory reputation for years since they were the first fats shown to increase levels of LDL (low-density lipoprotein, also known as "bad" cholesterol) and decrease levels of HDL (high-density lipoprotein, or "good" cholesterol), thus increasing the risk of heart disease. Dietary sources of saturated fats include meat, whole-milk dairy products, and egg yolks. Some plant foods such as coconut, palm, and palm kernel oils are also high in saturated fats. Saturated fats from any sources ought to be consumed sparingly, and limited to no more than 10 percent of your fat consumption.

Trans fats

In order to make polyunsaturated fats (PUFAs) that stay fresher longer, scientists have changed their chemical structure by infusing hydrogen gas so they remain solid at room temperature. Thus, the invention of partially hydrogenated vegetable oils that we know as trans fats.

Trans fats are the new "evil" fats because of a clear relationship between them and heart disease. Because of this established link, the U.S. Food and Drug Administration (FDA) now requires that products containing trans fats must declare them on the food label.

Many commercially baked goods (e.g., donuts, crackers, cookies) and processed/prepackaged products contain omega-6 fatty acids, especially partially hydrogenated ones (e.g., partially hydrogenated cottonseed oil). The way we prepare foods also influences their trans fat content. Foods fried in repeatedly heated vegetable oils (as is common practice in restaurants and fast-food establishments) are higher in trans fat than those fried in new oil. So those French fries from your favorite fast-food chain are a particularly unhealthy choice.

High glycemic index (GI) foods and inflammation

The rise in sugar consumption over the past century is another major nutrition change we have observed in our food industry. Sugar and foods that are made up of simple carbohydrates, also described as high GI foods, are associated with inflammation. GI is a measure of how much and how rapidly a food's carbohydrate content affects blood sugar levels after eating it. High GI foods include things like sugar-sweetened soda, candies (such as gum drops), and pasta and bread made from refined flour. Consuming too many high GI foods is linked to high blood sugar levels and insulin resistance. Higher insulin levels in response to our diets stimulate many parts of the inflammatory response.

Diets that are low in sugar and simple carbohydrates (low GI) have been shown to be associated with significantly less inflammation than diets that are low-fat but high in simple carbohydrates. Diets that emphasize monounsaturated fats, whole grains, lean meats and fish, fruits, and nuts (such as the "Mediterranean diet") are associated with less inflammation.

Fruits and vegetables and inflammation

Many studies have found a strong relationship between greater fruit and vegetable consumption and decreased risk of inflammation (lower C-reactive protein), as well as lower incidence of oxidative stress-driven conditions such as cardiovascular disease and cancer. This is because fruits and vegetables (especially red, orange, and yellow ones) are a rich source of antioxidants. During the weight-loss phase of the Medifast Program, it is important to incorporate high-antioxidant vegetables such as yellow peppers, spaghetti squash, tomatoes, broccoli, cauliflower, asparagus, and dark leafy greens. As you move into the Maintenance phase, you should gradually add high-antioxidant fruits such as berries, cherries, citrus fruits, papayas, and cantaloupe.

There are a few vegetables to be aware of if you are a person with food allergies. The nightshade vegetables, including eggplant, tomatoes, and potatoes, contain a chemical called solanine that may trigger an inflammatory response in some people.

Food preparation and inflammation

Overcooking our food can also increase inflammation. Overcooking or charring foods under the broiler or on the grill can lead to compounds called heat-generated advanced glycation end products (AGEs). These AGEs increase inflammation in the body, and have also been shown to increase LDL cholesterol. Food preparation practices like steaming or boiling are best for minimizing inflammation.

Antioxidants

Up to this point, we have learned that achieving and maintaining a healthy weight and eating the right foods can reduce the inflammation that leads to oxidative stress. Oxygen, while essential for life, also plays a part in the destruction of your body's tissues, impairing your organs' ability to function normally.[26] Every day, chemical reactions take place inside each tiny cell in your body. Oxidative stress in the body is a lot like rust on an old car. You can halt this "rusting" of your body by tackling free radicals.

Free radicals are products of normal cellular functioning, and may serve some biologic function, or they may simply be byproducts.[27] Free radicals are unstable, volatile molecules. Because they are missing an electron, they are highly reactive and seek to collide with other molecules so that they can "steal" electrons from molecules in healthy cells in an attempt to stabilize themselves. The healthy cells, once robbed, produce free radicals themselves, and a cycle begins. The multiplication of free radicals can lead to many different types of damage throughout the body.

Under normal conditions, a healthy body is able to defend itself against too many free radicals and maintain balance. But when we add other free radical-producing activities (e.g., smoking, drinking to excess, overeating), the additional free radical load may be too much for our body's normal systems to handle, and the wear-and-tear on our cells increases.

Oxidative stress compromises the ability of our cells' mitochondria (fat-burners) to function. This mitochondrial burnout, in turn, affects the ability of our cells our ability to transform food into energy. Extra food produces more free radicals, which overwhelm our natural antioxidant defense systems, leading to disease.

This is due to free radicals' high level of reactivity, which may indiscriminately damage cells' structure and function.[28] Although cells possess a variety of antioxidant defense mechanisms and repair systems, they can weaken as the high level of oxidative stress overwhelms their defenses.[28] Whether short- or long-term, this kind of cell stress has been blamed in a wide variety of human diseases, including diabetes, heart disease, cancer, and nervous system problems.[26]

Antioxidants prevent cell damage by replacing lost electrons in the molecules of cells throughout the body, replenishing electrons in the previously healthy cells, and strengthening impaired antioxidant defense systems. Antioxidants have many reported health benefits, including protecting and rejuvenating hair and skin cells, improving resistance to infection, increasing energy, and reducing the risk of coronary heart disease and cancer, as well as supporting healthy aging.

The antioxidant content of foods is expressed in oxygen radical absorbance capacity, or ORAC, value. In a study by the U.S. Department of Agriculture (USDA) Human Nutrition Research Center on Aging at Tufts University, men and women were asked to double their fruit and vegetable intake from an average of five servings of fruits and vegetables daily to 10. Before the study, the participants averaged 1,670 ORAC units daily based on questionnaire and diet data. Subjects who increased their fruit and vegetable servings to 10 a day raised their ORAC intake to between 3,300 and 3,500 ORAC units, or about twice the previous amount. Today, the USDA recommends an intake of 5,000 ORAC units per day to achieve optimum wellness. Sadly, 80 percent to 90 percent of us do not consume even half of that value.

You don't have to eat dozens of fruit and vegetable servings each day to get the recommended amounts of antioxidants. With a little knowledge, you can concentrate on foods that offer the most antioxidants for the mouthful. The following tables (Tables 4 and 5) show the ORAC values of antioxidant-rich foods and herbs to include in your diet.[29] You will be surprised to find that many foods and herbs you may already have in your own home have a high ORAC level.

Vegetables

Make sure to include the following "Green" options with high ORAC values as part of your weight-loss plan:

Table 4. "Green" options antioxidant power[29]

Vegetables	ORAC units per 100 grams
Lettuce, *green leaf, raw*	2,380
Radishes, *raw*	1,736
Spinach, *frozen*	1,687
Asparagus, *cooked, boiled*	1,644
Red onions, *raw*	1,521
Broccoli, *raw*	1,362
Green bell peppers, *raw*	923
Orange peppers, *raw*	984
Cauliflower, *boiled*	829

Herbs and spices

Herbs and spices are a great way to add flavor to your food and creativity to your cooking, and several of your favorite herbs also contain beneficial anti-inflammatory, antioxidant compounds. Use the following anti-inflammatory herbs and spices to flavor your meals and boost your ORAC score, and remember to stick to the serving sizes that keep you compliant with your phase of the Medifast Program.

Table 5. Antioxidant-rich herbs and spices[29]

Herbs	ORAC units per 1 gram
Cloves	3,144
Cinnamon	2,675
Oregano	2,001
Turmeric *(ground)*	1,593
Parsley	743
Curry powder	485
Sage	320
Ginger	288
Thyme	274
Chili powder	236

Tea

Tea is more than just a tasty, invigorating beverage. To varying degrees, white, green, and black teas all contain antioxidants called catechins. White tea contains the greatest amount, followed by green and black. The ORAC value of brewed black tea is 1,128 and that of brewed green tea is 1,362. The less the tea has been processed or fermented, the higher the antioxidant content. White and green teas are minimally processed, and thus yield the highest amount of antioxidants.

Dark chocolate

Chocolate lovers will be glad to know that dark chocolate is a healthy part of an anti-inflammatory diet (when consumed in moderation and during the Maintenance phase of your program). The catechins in dark chocolate are rich with antioxidant properties, especially dark chocolate that is made from 70 percent cocoa. Dark chocolate contains roughly 10 times more catechins and antioxidant activity than milk chocolate. Even when you're in the weight-loss phase and you're not indulging in chocolate candy, Medifast's Dark Chocolate Shake is an enjoyable way to get the antioxidants—and taste—of dark chocolate throughout your weight-loss or maintenance program.

Essential1: Antioxidants

To ensure you reach your optimal intake of antioxidants, Medifast has formulated both Essential1: Antioxidants Shakes and Essential1: Antioxidants Flavor Infusers™ as a front-line defense against free radicals and oxidative stress. Each Shake and Flavor Infuser™ has an ORAC value of 1,000 and was designed to promote:

- Control of free radicals
- Cardiovascular health
- Optimal brain function and mental acuity
- Clear vision
- Healthy aging process
- Balanced blood sugar levels
- Urinary tract health.

In addition to 1,000 ORAC units, each Essential1: Antioxidants Flavor Infuser™ provides 15 mg of resveratrol. Resveratrol, an antioxidant in red wine, has received a lot of media attention recently for its ability to extend lifespan in animal models.[30] When given to yeast cells, fruit flies, worms, and mice, resveratrol extends the average lifespan by 70 percent. Like these lower life forms, humans have a "survival gene" that activates an enzyme system that improves mitochondrial conversion of nutrients into energy, insulin sensitivity, and exercise endurance. That means resveratrol may be particularly appropriate for individuals who are obese or who have diabetes, as some studies have found these individuals have smaller, less well-functioning mitochondria, resulting in problems converting nutrients into energy.

Resveratrol has also been shown to have a broad range of health-enhancing properties, including anti-oxidant, anti-inflammatory, and anti-microbial bacterial actions. It has been shown to suppress tumor cells; improve disease states such as cardiovascular disease, cancer, and diabetes; and combat infections of the stomach like *Helicobacter pylori*, a bacterium associated with ulcers and other digestive diseases.

Many scientists speculate that resveratrol in red wine is responsible for what's known as the "French Paradox." Despite consuming a diet rich in fatty foods, the French have lower rates of heart disease, and doctors have wondered if this is due to the antioxidants in the red wine that the French so often enjoy along with those rich foods. Since alcoholic beverages are not part of our weight-loss plan, Essential1: Antioxidants Flavor Infusers™ provide a way to get a healthy amount of resveratrol—even better than a glass of red wine with dinner. In fact, just one serving contains as much resveratrol as 16 bottles of red wine, and the same amount of antioxidants as in two pieces of fruit—but without the alcohol, sugar, or calories.

After reading this chapter, you should now understand that reducing inflammation and oxidative stress by decreasing your body fat (especially around the middle) and through eating anti-inflammatory foods well can move you ahead on your pathway to health. As you lose and maintain your weight, remember to include omega-3 fatty acids, resveratrol, and low GI, antioxidant-rich foods, while avoiding too much saturated fat, trans fat, and sugar. Doing so will help ease the process of aging, and lessen your risk for inflammatory conditions like heart disease and certain cancers.

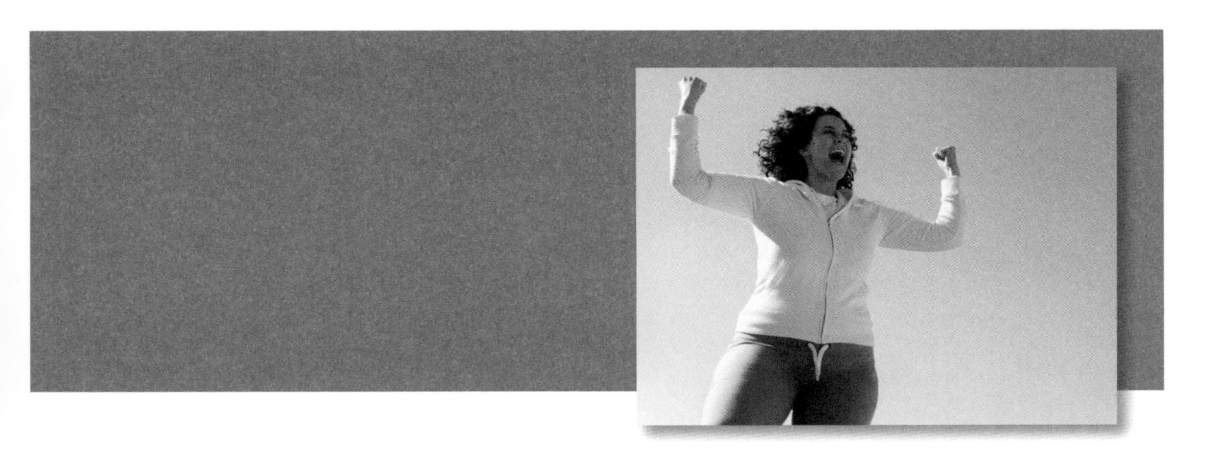

5 Personal journey

Getting into the Medifast mind set

Now that you are aware of some of the larger external forces at hand, like the fat-promoting environment, and the fundamental flaws of other diets and why they have failed you, it is time to turn your focus inward. Before beginning the Medifast Program, you must get into the mind-set that you will succeed. You must remember that the most valuable resource you have in weight loss and in life is you. Fighting for your health may be one of the most important things you do. You may be fighting to see your grandchildren grow up. Or fighting to play more with your children. Or fighting to spend more years with your spouse. But the most important thing you're fighting for is you. There's nothing more self-defeating than the endless merry-go-round of weight loss and weight gain. It can stop today and Medifast can help.

Get committed

Probably one of the easiest aspects of the Medifast Program is eating the pre-packaged, nutritionally enhanced Medifast Meals. They taste good and are easy to keep on-hand. The harder part of following the plan will be overcoming some of the outside obstacles you will face. In order to beat the challenges that lie ahead, you are going to have to make some major commitments.

Commitment 1: I will comply with the Medifast program and consume only the products allowed until I have reached my goal weight.

Commitment 2: I will make changes in my eating habits and change my old beliefs about dieting.

Commitment 3: I will include an exercise program and record my activity.

Commitment 4: I will be honest with myself about the troubles I am having and will get the support I need. Whether it is through Medifast, a support group, or a special person, I will be accountable to someone.

These commitments won't be easy. But you can do it. Remember, the most valuable resource you've got is you!

You don't have to make food choices, you don't have to worry about calories, and you'll lose weight without feeling particularly hungry or deprived. You will likely look and feel better than you have in years, maybe your entire life! But you will be faced with the same urges and pressures to eat that have plagued you on other diets. We live in a fat-promoting, food-oriented society, and just about every social activity centers on food. You'll find temptations everywhere. But when you have the right motivation for success, trust in yourself, and belief that your health is worth fighting for, you will succeed.

Set reasonable goals

Now that you are committed, you need to set reasonable goals. You may be asking, "Why should I have goals?," or "What are goals anyway?," or "Are goals really necessary?" Understanding goals will help you understand the Medifast Program and incorporate the tools you need to achieve lasting success.

Goals are priorities. They are commitments that you make to yourself. They are your decisions about where you are in your life and where you want to be. For example, if your doctor said you need to maintain a certain weight for good health and you are 10 pounds above that weight, your goal will be to lose those 10 pounds.

How do you identify your goals? At the surface, you need to ask yourself why you want to lose weight. Is it to look good for someone else? To attend a class reunion? To be thin for your daughter's wedding? These types of goals are considered short-term goals and don't usually last. When you are motivated by short-term success, it's too easy to lose interest and enthusiasm.

You have to ask yourself what you—no one else but you—want for your life. Do you want a lifetime of good health? Do you want to live longer for your children and grandchildren? These are things you need to decide before you start setting your goals. Be mindful of your goals. Know exactly what you want for yourself to keep your focus sharp and your motivation strong.

Put your goals down on paper. Keep them in a place that is close to you—your wallet, by your bed, in your car, on your refrigerator. Somewhere you will see them: They'll remind you of whom and what you are working for. Avoid words like "should," "ought to," "never," and "always." These words will set you up for failure. Always stay positive.

It's best to keep goals small, positive, and attainable because it allows you to achieve small successes and stay motivated.

What are my personal goals?

In order to determine what your personal weight loss goals should be, you'll want to identify what experts consider to be an appropriate body weight for your height. The following table may give you a sense of what your weight loss target should be. Note that the higher weights generally apply to men (who tend to have more muscle and bone) and the lower weights more often apply to women (who have less muscle and bone).

Table 1. Suggested weights for adults.

Height *(without shoes)*	Weight in lbs *(with little to no clothing)*	
	19 to 34 years old	*35 years and over*
5′0″	97-128	108-138
5′1″	101-132	111-143
5′2″	104-137	115-148
5′3″	107-141	119-152
5′4″	111-146	122-157
5′5″	114-150	126-162
5′6″	118-155	130-167
5′7″	121-160	134-172
5′8″	125-164	138-178
5′9″	129-169	142-183
5′10″	132-174	146-188
5′11″	136-179	151-194
6′0″	140-184	155-199
6′1″	144-189	159-205
6′2″	148-195	164-210
6′3″	152-200	168-216
6′4″	156-205	173-222
6′5″	160-211	177-228
6′6″	164-216	182-234

Source: Derived from the National Research Council, 1989. http://www.nal.usda.gov/fnic/dga/resource.htm

Instead of body weight, you may prefer to monitor your success through clothing sizes, with a tape measure, or by another method. Just remember that you do not have to be perfect. Any amount of weight loss is progress. If you expect perfection, you will be disappointed and set yourself up for failure. No one can ever be perfect all of the time.

Before you begin a program of healthy living—a program that's going to require you to change habits and break old patterns—it's important to take a hard look at why you want to lose weight. You have to give these reasons careful thought and consideration. It's equally important to write them down.

These personal goals have to be about what you want for yourself—not what other people say you should do or what you think other people expect of you. Avoid using negatives when setting goals. "I don't want to be fat anymore" is self-defeating. Positive momentum is what will keep you going.

Take a minute and think about what matters to you most. Is it spending time with your family? Sitting on the beach? Improving your health? Some people find health an abstract reason, so it is important to personalize it—such as, "I want to lower my blood pressure because I want to enjoy my retirement with my spouse," or "I want to lower my cholesterol because I want to see my children graduate from college." Everyone is different, and your goals need to be personal so you'll keep them.

Take a few moments each day to thoughtfully read through your list. Make a promise to yourself now, "I will read through this list when I am confronted with a difficult food decision, or when I'm tired and frustrated and want to quit. I will read through this list because I'm making a commitment to the most important person I know—me." Reading through the list will reinforce your commitment to yourself to take control of your health and self-esteem.

How do I achieve my goals?

You've likely come to realize that while some goals may seem daunting on the surface, they become much easier to attain once they're broken down into small, easy-to-accomplish steps. When organized properly, the time and energy required to reach your goals decreases significantly. Here are a few hints:

- Monitor your progress on at least a weekly basis. Studies indicate that frequent, regular self-monitoring is a predictor of success in weight control. Know what you have accomplished and be aware of what needs to be done.
- Give yourself non-food rewards like some extra time reading a book, a longer call to a friend, or a bouquet of flowers for yourself. Reward

10 Reasons Why I Want To Lose Weight

1. ____

2. ____

3. ____

4. ____

5. ____

6. ____

7. ____

8. ____

9. ____

10. ____

**Take special note of your top two reasons for wanting to lose weight. They can be particularly insightful.*

yourself for a job well done.

- Honest self-assessment and behavior modification are keys to achieving goals. You must become aware of the problem areas in your life and be willing to make changes. There are no quick fixes for weight management.
- Keep goals simple—don't make a goal so complex that you have to try and figure out what you are trying to do.
- Make goals realistic—don't underestimate your capabilities or overstate your capacities.

Be practical when it comes to expectations

What kind of weight loss can you expect? Many variables factor into the amount of weight you can anticipate losing on Medifast. A lot depends on your metabolism. Your age and gender play an important role in determining your metabolism, as do things that you can change such as the amount of muscle mass you have. Even certain medications can impact your weight-loss efforts. Your rate of weight loss will also vary depending on if you are in the initial phase of the plan or in the final phase, near your goal weight.

> If you are sticking to your plan faithfully, there's nothing you can do to make the weight loss go any faster than it's going to go.

So, it's best to think of weight loss and good health as a 26-mile marathon rather than a 50-yard dash. You're in this for the long haul and Medifast is there with you, every step of the way.

Weight loss can be significant during the initial phase of Medifast. Some may lose five to seven pounds (or more) per week. Most everyone ends their first week with significant weight loss. Some of this is water weight. The general rule of thumb when it comes to Medifast is that most people tend to lose about two to five pounds per week, or up to 20 pounds in 30 days.

If you find the scale discouraging, then use a tape measure. Tape measurements aren't influenced by fluid changes as much as the scale is, and therefore can more accurately reflect your results. Some people use the same pair of pants. Trying the same pair on week after week will show you that the weight is coming off and will give you the encouragement to keep going.

You may be wondering what happens once you reach your goal weight and begin eating regular food again. There are three things you need to be aware of.

First, if you lose a significant amount of weight, say over 20 pounds, some weight will come back initially. Don't panic. The increased sodium and carbohydrates you're eating again may cause you to retain water. You are not on your way to gaining fat weight. As your body adjusts to regular food again, so will your scale.

Second, your metabolism slows down on the Medifast Program and it will take a month or two to speed up again. When your metabolism slows down, you are burning fewer calories and need to take a careful look at your food intake and exercise level. For this reason, the Medifast Program has you reintroduce regular food slowly to minimize the effect of these changes on metabolism.

Last, when you reach your goal weight, you need to understand that you cannot go back to eating the way you did prior to Medifast. That's how you gained weight in the first place. Medifast gives you food plans for healthy living. Yes, you will always have to watch what you eat because every healthy person does. But that doesn't mean a lifetime of sacrifice and starvation. It means caring for yourself like you do for your garden, your car, or your house. You need to listen to your body and monitor your health. You don't put gas in your car every time you feel sad, go to a party, or are out with your friends. You only put gas in your car when the tank is empty. It's the same with your body. Eat when you're hungry and eat what makes you run well for a lifetime of good health.

> Prior to starting Medifast, we strongly recommend that you keep a food record of what you normally eat in a given week. Every bite, every cracker, every sip of your child's juice, every spoonful of ice cream counts. Remember, this is designed to help you see what you do before you start your weight-loss program. At the end of the week, take a look. It is helpful to get out a calorie counter and take a look at the actual number of calories. It can be frightening. But in the end, it can help you realize how you got where you are and then empower you to make the changes you need for long-term success.

Identify your food cues and counteract them

Many overweight people say they don't know how they gained the weight. They eat a healthy dinner, they eat breakfast, they eat a salad for lunch. Yet the scale keeps creeping upward and the button on their pants keeps getting harder and harder to close. Snacks in the office lunch room ... appetizers at a friend's after work ... dinner out ... a cookie here ... a soda there ... It all adds up. And most of us don't even realize what's happening until it's too late. So let's get familiar with how the weight crept on. To control your eating, you need to be aware of what your eating cues are. When you anticipate situations before they occur, you can troubleshoot.

Stress

Have you ever sat down and asked, "What is making me eat so much?" Many researchers would probably say stress. It's important to figure out what is stressing you out. Often it's because you're not able to meet some of your basic needs. Your personal and professional lives determine your basic needs. Stress in these areas can wreak havoc on your life. Overeating in response to stress is a negative coping mechanism.

The Solution

Use positive coping mechanisms as a way to de-stress (e.g. yoga, exercise). These mechanisms can also be therapeutic.

The workplace

The workplace is a major source of stress in our world today. How many of us have gone home after a tough day at work and eaten everything in sight? Unfortunately, most of us can't afford to give up working, so we need to find ways to reduce the stress at work. Poor communication between coworkers and bosses can be an enormous source of stress. Feeling like you are the only one that can get the job done right and doing all the work yourself can also add to the burden.

The Solution

At work, if you find that you run around all day but never get anything done, maybe you need to practice better time management. Getting organized and making priorities can go a long way to reduce stress at work. Trying to communicate your needs and clarify the needs of others will help this problem. Why not try delegating responsibilities and give others a chance to prove themselves? If the job has become routine or boring, develop creative ways to get the work done. If all these fail, motivate yourself to look for a new job.

Loneliness

Everyone needs relationships with other people. The most obvious sources are your friends and family, but what do you do if you don't have close friends or family?

The Solution

If you are lonely, meeting people with similar interests can generate lifelong friendships. Try joining volunteer organizations, hobby clubs, hiking groups, or bike clubs. Or you might take an educational course to meet other people.

Boredom

It's amazing how, with nothing else to do, our thoughts turn to food. With nothing better to do, we often find ourselves in the kitchen checking out the fridge or cupboards. But this form of eating has nothing to do with hunger, and everything to do with keeping ourselves occupied.

The Solution

Get busy. Have you ever noticed that the busier you are, the less you think about food? One of the best ways to control eating is to fill your day with activities that aren't synonymous with eating. Instead of eating, why not walk your dog or offer to walk your neighbor's dog? Start a new hobby like gardening, knitting, or golfing that will keep your hands busy and away from your mouth. Go out and buy a gift for someone you love, or pick a flower from your garden and put it in a vase. You may wind up discovering talents you didn't know you had!

Peer pressure

In social settings, peer pressure can play a large role in eating and drinking. Friends will often encourage us to "have another drink, it's Friday night!" But is the arrival of Friday night really such a big deal?

The Solution

Surround yourself with supportive friends. Don't be afraid to tell friends and family how they can help you stick with your plan, and confront those who are intentionally or unintentionally sabotaging your efforts.

Comfort

After an awful day at work or following a fight with your partner, family member, or friend, it can feel as though you really deserve some enjoyable food—whether you are hungry or not. Unfortunately, comfort eating can have the complete opposite effect from the one you were hoping to achieve. We often eat to cheer ourselves up, but then we remember that we shouldn't be eating and feel even worse than before. Since we feel even worse, we are driven to eat more in hopes of feeling good again (at least temporarily). You can see how this cycle becomes a vicious one.

The Solution

Find alternative ways to comfort yourself—a walk, a bath, a book, a small (non-food) present to yourself.

Helpful hints when it comes to inappropriate eating

Pre-plan your approach so you can head off inappropriate eating and eating binges.

No two people are the same. You need to figure out what works best for you. Write down what your eating cues and trouble spots are, then devise a game plan to avoid or deal with those trouble spots without resorting to food. For example, you may decide to stay away from certain fast-food establishments by taking a slightly different route home from work.

Control your environment before it controls you.

Keep a "healthy" house. Your environment can be an eating trigger. Junk food in the house can be a major cue for food cravings. There is an important distinction between the psychological desire for food (craving) and the physiological need for food (hunger). Craving is the desire for food even though your body doesn't need the extra nourishment. Craving can be caused by smelling fresh cookies in the oven or sizzling bacon on the stove, or by just thinking about food. You only experience true hunger when your body actually needs nourishment. This doesn't happen until you haven't eaten for an extended period of time. It can produce a gnawing sensation in the stomach, light-headedness, headache, irritability, or lethargy. If you're like most people, your overeating has been the result of psychological urges to eat.

We often give in to our cravings, so if high-calorie foods aren't kept in the house, we can't eat them. And fortunately, all food cravings ultimately pass! The truth is that no one requires high-calorie junk foods (including children and spouses), and most of us could stand to develop better eating habits. If family members insist on griping, get them to buy their own single-serving snacks. Defend yourself and your weight-loss efforts. You've earned it.

Designate one area as your eating area.

If you find yourself eating everywhere in the house, create one space just for eating. This makes you get up and go somewhere when you want to snack, and it makes you more aware of eating patterns. Eating while standing in the kitchen, watching television, driving, or talking on the phone is mindless eating. Pay attention to what, when, and where you are eating.

Reduce your visual cues.

Reduce the temptation of junk food by not buying it in the first place. If it is in the house, put it out of sight. Remove all food containers and serving bowls from the table. Don't automatically take a second helping. Vow never to eat on the way to the sink, standing up, off your children's plate, or on the way to the trash can.

Watch out for time cues.

Weekends

The weekend is here, it's time to eat! A study published in the August 2003 issue of Obesity Research found that American adults took in 115 more calories per day on the weekend (defined as Friday through Sunday) than on other days of the week. While that might not sound so bad, the problem is that it can really add up over time. Over the course of a year, that adds up to 17,940 extra calories—or about five pounds gained. As you might suspect, the 115-calorie-a-day difference comes mostly from fat and alcohol.

Holidays

Thanksgiving is our favorite holiday for eating. It is commonly believed that the average American will gain five to seven pounds during the holidays. The good news is that the average weight gain is only one pound, according to the National Institute of Diabetes and Digestive and Kidney Diseases (NIDDK). The bad news is that many people are not shedding the excess weight after the holidays, and those extra pounds add up over time.

Special occasions

This ties into holiday eating, but for some people, special occasions come around quite often—for instance, every Saturday night in the bar, every time football is on TV, or every time they've conquered the house cleaning.

Spectator eating

For many of us, a bucket of popcorn at the movies or a bowl of tortilla chips on the coffee table during a football game are part of the viewing experience. Eating while engrossed in something else (e.g., reading a book, working on the computer, writing an essay) is an easy way to eat much more than you intended. At the end of the movie or the end of the game, it's easy to look down and see that the entire bucket of popcorn or bowl of chips has been eaten without you even noticing. This is a waste of calories at best.

Watch out for saboteurs—identifying weight-loss friends and foes

Losing weight and getting healthy is one of the most positive things we can do for ourselves. However, behavior changes can be frightening (and difficult) for us and those around us.

Family and friend sabotage is one of the most frequently overlooked and misunderstood factors in our current overweight epidemic. Self-defeating attitudes and behaviors often drive us to act against our desire to be healthy. If that were not bad enough, sometimes our friends and family want us to stay the same, and their behavior can create obstacles not easily seen or solved. In fact, many times those around us inflict their beliefs and insecurities on us.

How do you know if there's a saboteur in your midst? Sometimes they're obvious and sometimes they're virtually invisible. Unfortunately there's no radar screen you can scan that would reveal the hostile blips in your zone, but you can usually identify saboteurs by monitoring their behavior.

What do saboteurs around you do when you try to lose weight? There's a long list of red flags. Some common sabotage tactics include criticizing, withdrawing, becoming overly involved (or under-involved) in your weight loss efforts, or erecting other obstacles. Any time another's behavior gets in the way of your success, there's a good chance sabotage is at work.

Why would someone act this way? The simplest answer is that a saboteur may actually want you to remain overweight. For example, your partner feels less threatened about rejection or abandonment as long as you are overweight. Or, your weight problem serves as a convenient distraction from other problems in the relationship, so there's motivation for your weight to hang around. Finally, your partner or friends may be unmotivated to address their own weight problem. Feeling shamed by your success, they do things to derail your efforts.

Because social support is a key ingredient to changing any behavior, it is important to assess your personal network when you plan lifestyle modifications. Who are the genuine sources of support, and who are not? If or when you identify saboteurs, your strategy then depends on the type of saboteur you're up against. Can the saboteur be changed or avoided? Often, the solution lies in confronting this person and communicating your needs. If that doesn't work, protect yourself from this person's negativity, so that you don't lose sight of what you're trying to accomplish.

Be aware that when we make changes to ourselves, those around us may have difficulty accepting those changes. Losing weight is hard enough as it is, avoiding saboteurs is one way to make it easier. Here's a short list of tips for handling saboteurs:

1. Tune in to your support network and identify true friends and foes.
2. Communicate your needs.
3. Be forthright and persistent in stating your requests.
4. Avoid or limit time with saboteurs who won't change their ways.
5. Keep focused on your personal goals.
6. Seek support from others facing similar weight challenges.

Perfectionism

If you fall off the weight-loss wagon, get right back up there. Don't expect to be a perfect dieter. So very few of us are. Instead of setting the bar so high that failure is likely, be realistic and build some relapses into your plan. That way, if you fall off the wagon you won't beat yourself up about it. You'll know what to do—get started again.

Very few people associate perfectionism with being overweight, but it's true. Most people who are overweight struggle with perfectionism. If they can't do a diet perfectly, they go back to their old ways.

Perfectionism is not a healthy pursuit of excellence. There are big differences between perfectionists and healthy achievers. Perfectionists believe that mistakes must never be made and that the highest standards of performance must always be achieved. Those who strive for excellence in a healthy way take genuine pleasure in trying to meet high standards. Perfectionists on the other hand are full of self-doubt. They fear disapproval, ridicule, and rejection. The healthy striver has drive, while the perfectionist is driven.

Perfectionism is:

- The irrational belief that you and/or your environment must be perfect.
- An all-pervasive attitude that whatever you attempt in life must be done letter perfect with no deviation, mistakes, slip ups, or inconsistencies.
- A habit developed from youth that keeps you constantly alert to the imperfections, failings, and weaknesses in yourself and others.
- The underlying motive present in the fear of failure and fear of rejection (e.g., if I am not perfect, I will fail, I will be rejected by others).
- A reason why you may be fearful of success (e.g., if I achieve my goal, will I be able to continue/maintain that level of achievement?).
- The belief that no matter what you attempt, it is never good enough to meet your own or others' expectations.

Examples of the negative consequences of perfectionism

Low self-esteem. A perfectionist never feels good enough about personal performance; therefore, feelings of being a failure or a loser (with a lessening of self-confidence and self-esteem) may result.

Guilt. Because a perfectionist never feels good about the way responsibility has been handled in life (by himself or others) feelings of shame, self recrimination, and guilt may result.

Pessimism. Since a perfectionist is convinced that it will be extremely difficult to achieve an *ideal goal*, he can easily become discouraged, fatalistic, disheartened, and pessimistic about future efforts to reach a goal.

Depression. Needing always to be perfect (yet recognizing that it is impossible to achieve such a goal) a perfectionist runs the risk of feeling down, blue, and depressed.

Rigidity. Needing to have everything in one's life perfect or *just so* can lead a perfectionist to an extreme case of being inflexible, non-spontaneous, and rigid.

Obsessiveness. Being in need of an excessive amount of order, pattern, or structure in life can lead a perfectionist to become nit-picky, finicky, or obsessive in an effort to maintain a certain order.

Compulsive behavior. Over-indulgence or the compulsive use of alcohol, drugs, gambling, food, shopping, sex, smoking, risk-taking, or novelty, is often used to medicate a perfectionist who feels like a failure or loser for never being able to be *good enough* in life.

Lack of motivation. Believing that the goal of change can never be ideally or perfectly achieved, can often give a perfectionist a lack of motivation to attempt change in the first place, or to persevere if change has already begun.

Immobilization. Because a perfectionist is often burdened with an extreme fear of failure, the person can become immobilized. With no energy, effort, or creative juices applied to rectify, improve, or change problem behaviors, the perfectionist becomes stagnant.

Lack of belief in oneself. Knowing that one will never be able to achieve an idyllic goal can lead a perfectionist to lose the belief that he will ever be able to improve his life significantly.

But there is hope. Many people have been able to lose weight and overcome perfectionism. But there are some critical steps you have to take.

Acceptance. No one is perfect, and being a perfectionist is a very difficult way to live. It is far better to accept yourself for who you are. The pressure of trying to be perfect has a significant impact on your health and your relationships. Try to stop being critical of yourself and others and allow some room for error. This does not mean you should not strive to improve yourself, only that you must be reasonable in your goals and expectations. Begin to revel in the joy of being on the journey of life with the rest of us.

Forgiveness. We all need forgiveness. While it sounds like a cliché, it's often hardest to simply forgive ourselves. Looking at the world through a negative prism robs you of the joy of living. No wonder you turn to food for comfort. You're always mad at yourself for one thing or another. Today is the day to stop being angry with yourself for whatever you feel you've done wrong and start getting with healthy living.

Starting over. So you have a bad eating day. One bad day doesn't have to turn into another. Pick yourself up, dust yourself off, and get back on your weight-loss plan. Look forward, not backward.

No one can be perfect or even eat healthy all the time. Medifast is a program for real people. It's okay if you slip. Life isn't perfect and neither are we. It's easier to live that way. Enjoy your imperfections and those of the people you love. It's what makes you who you are.

Patience. Develop a sense of patience with yourself and others. Setting unrealistic or unreasonable goals is a recipe for disaster. Backsliding does not mean the end of the world. With your renewed good health you should have a long and productive life. That life will include occasional (or frequent) backsliding. You don't have to be a superstar. No one really is. We all have our faults and most of the people we know are well aware of them. Try to enjoy being human and let go of the idea of ever being super-human. It's too hard and it takes time away from enjoying those we love.

Contrary to what most of us think, healthy living starts from the inside. We have to let go of the "shoulds" in our lives and learn to enjoy who we are. We can appreciate our achievements with a healthy sense of pride, as opposed to false humility and self-deprecation.

If you have led a lifetime of yo-yo dieting and setbacks, it's now time to reward yourself for the successes in your life, no matter how small. One day of healthy eating should be seen as an accomplishment.

Start to reward yourself for your progress. Learn to be flexible in goal setting. The most important thing is to realize that you're moving in a positive direction after perhaps many years of setbacks.

The last 10 pounds

Anyone who's ever dieted knows those last 10 pounds are usually the hardest to lose. At this point maybe you're tired and ready to go back to regular eating. Or you're asking yourself how important are these silly last few pounds anyway? Or worse, you're afraid that once you reach that final goal you won't be able to keep the weight off and you'll be back to the races again. Even if you've lost some initial weight relatively easy, the last 10 pounds can be the hardest to lose because for so many years you've been yo-yo dieting. 10 pounds down, 20 pounds up. You've gotten so discouraged that even you don't believe in yourself anymore. Maybe you're afraid that once you reach your goal you won't be able to keep the weight off again. But we know if you've gotten this far, you're capable of setting your mind to something and sticking to it.

So how do you stay motivated to reach your final goal and stay there afterwards? Remember to begin with small goals that are easy to achieve. During the first few weeks on the Medifast program you may have lost three or more pounds a week, and now you're down to one or two a week. Not a problem, and not unexpected. Any weight lost is a win for you. Try telling yourself that this week, "I'll try a little harder," or "I'll exercise just a little bit more," or "I'll take the stairs a few more times and avoid the elevator."

Remember to stick to your goals. With the goal weight in sight and the introduction of regular grocery food, it's easy to let cheating creep back in. Be good to yourself and your commitments by sticking to the program. You deserve all your success and should keep focusing on the goal of good health.

Some people love the attention they receive from a new physique. They get a big boost of self-esteem when receiving compliments from family and friends. Others find it uncomfortable at first. If you've been heavy for a while all the new attention can be unsettling. Take the compliments as a job well done and revel in your success.

Make lasting changes

To lose weight successfully you have to change the way you think about things. You may not realize that the way you think about things has a great impact on your ability to lose weight and sustain the loss. Weight management isn't as simple as just watching what you eat. Otherwise you wouldn't be reading this book! Change involves motivation, goals, and learning how to best deal with mistakes.

Our thoughts have a powerful influence over our behavior. In fact, our thoughts are often transferred directly to behavior. For example, if you think that keeping a food record is a pain and takes too much time, the resulting behavior is that you don't keep records. On the other hand, if you change your thinking, you can change your behavior. If you think that keeping a food record only takes a small amount of time and will help you lose weight, then you will keep the food record.

Your self-image—how you see yourself—is a mirror of your thoughts. Your self-image reflects the actions you take, the goals you will set and be able to keep, and how you picture or label yourself. As we know all too well, when you weigh too much your self-image is often poor. You feel worthless and unattractive because you can't control your eating. Starting the Medifast Program is a positive action that reflects your desire to make changes and lose weight for good. That's a great step, and you're heading in the right direction to improve your life.

But simply losing weight may not change your self-esteem. That's why so many people experience the "yo-yo" effect of weight loss and weight gain. Why? Because many people hold onto old beliefs about themselves. How can you improve your self-image? First develop a new definition of yourself. You are not your weight problem. It is helpful here to write down all of your good characteristics and start emphasizing them. Work to develop new skills. Try things you've always wanted to try (but were too afraid to). Each success will lead to improved self-esteem.

Asserting yourself in a positive way at work or at home can also have a positive effect on your self-esteem. When you don't let your feelings and opinions be known, you feel that others are taking advantage of you. Many overweight people feel that they are invisible. It's important to learn how to stand up for yourself without hurting others. Fear of hurting others and losing approval is often what causes people to keep their feelings and opinions to themselves.

Beliefs can have a tremendous impact on weight-loss efforts. Many of us have said things like, "I'm too heavy to exercise," or "I have no will power," or "I was a fat child and I will always be fat," or "My metabolism is too slow for me to lose weight." Faulty beliefs are often used as justification for not making positive changes. You take on the attitude that you can't do certain things, and then you don't even try. You use the beliefs as a way to say I don't have to exercise, lose weight, or change my eating habits. This too can change.

Positive beliefs are critical for weight-loss success. "I have to start slow, but I can exercise," "I have the power to control my eating habits," "I was an overweight child but I don't have to be an overweight adult," and "I will stay with the weight-loss program even if the weight loss is slow," are examples of beliefs that encourage action. They are realistic and will create an environment that will lead to positive change.

Once beliefs change, positive actions become the norm. You establish a regular exercise routine that you can stick to. You identify cues to eating and develop controls. You take the steps you need to lose weight and make the changes to keep the weight off for good.

Self-image and belief work together to control your thoughts. If you incorporate an improved self-image with positive beliefs, you will create new thoughts. It will be these new thoughts that determine your new behaviors. The end result is worth the effort.

Behavior changes don't occur by thought alone. You have to believe in the changes you make and you have to plan for changes that will help you achieve your goals. If you want to change your eating habits, you need to make a sincere effort, and you will need to direct your efforts towards a specific and realistic goal.

Be mindful—how to eat healthy for life

So far, this chapter focused on developing healthy belief systems and behavioral tactics for weight control. Now this chapter will advise you how to eat foods. Medifast recommends a "mindful" approach to the way you eat foods. Being mindful about food simply means being consciously aware on a moment-to-moment basis about the food you eat, the process of eating that food, and how the food makes your body feel. By paying attention to the food you eat and your body's response to eating it, several positive things happen:

- You gain control over the food.
- You learn how to distinguish feelings of hunger from feelings of emptiness, or any other reason why you may be eating.
- You learn how to form a positive relationship with food. Appreciate all of the qualities the food has to offer (e.g., flavor, texture). This requires eating slowly and savoring each bite. Appreciating food in this way helps you to eat less. In return, foods will be good to you by keeping you healthy and slim.
- You learn how to tune in with your hunger level and how it decreases with each bite of food. Eating slowly and mindfully, cues you into feelings of fullness sooner than when eating on auto-pilot.

Tips on how to eat mindfully

Tip #1

Mindful eating involves a little planning. Overeating can begin before food ever touches your lips. That's because we make choices about food when we go grocery shopping, or when we order dinner in a restaurant. Deciding to *treat* yourself at the grocery store or restaurant is an act of planning to overeat. So, make a shopping list before you go to the grocery store, or decide what you are going to order and how much of it you plan to eat while out at a restaurant.[31]

Tip #2

Once the food is in front of you, mindfully approach it by taking a minute or so to think about the food you are planning to eat before jumping right in. In other words, don't take the food for granted just because it is there. Remember to give it the respect it deserves by appreciating the way the food looks and how it smells. Then, take a few deep breaths before you sit down at the table. This will help you approach the food mindfully.[31]

Tip #3

Cut your food up into small pieces. Once you begin to eat, pay attention to all the qualities the food has to offer. Then take a small bite of food and chew it slowly, at least 20 times before swallowing. Think about the current bite of food in your mouth, focusing on its specific qualities (e.g., taste, texture, mouth feel). After you have swallowed it, then you can begin to think about taking the next bite. Repeat this process for each bite of food you eat. This technique will be especially helpful as you enjoy the tasty but smaller portions of Medifast foods.[31]

Tip #4

While you are eating, there are some tricks that will help you slow down and appreciate each bite of food. The first trick is to take a bite of food then put your fork or spoon down. Chew slowly and savor the food. Repeat with each bite of food. In the case of a flavored beverage (e.g., Medifast Shake), take a sip and put it down. Savor the taste of the drink. Another trick is to take a sip of water between each bite of food or sip of flavored beverage (e.g., Medifast Shake). This helps you appreciate the unique qualities of the food or beverage.[31]

Tip #5

After mindfully eating your first few bites of food, tune into your feelings of hunger and ask yourself, "Am I still hungry?" Food cravings and hunger pangs are generally alleviated after the first few bites of food. You can do your own experiment to check and see. Take a Medifast bar, for instance. See if the gratification you feel after the tenth bite is truly as gratifying as the first. The likelihood is that while indeed the bar still tastes good, the gratification feels less intense. Simply put, the "ahhh" sensation you get with the first bite or two of food becomes less and less as you eat. So the trick is to focus on the first few bites of food and savor them. Continue to eat after that point only if truly hungry. This will satisfy the fix you are seeking with far fewer calories.[31]

Tip #6

Be mindful of what appropriate portions are. Create visual borders on your plate to help you be mindful of your portions. You can do this by visualizing your plate as having a central region and an outside region. The center is your region of interest. Cut up your food into tiny pieces, then separate it by moving half of each type of food to the center region of your plate, and half of it to the outside region (or edges) of your plate. Focus on eating the food in the center of your plate first. Eat it mindfully. Ask yourself, "Am I still hungry?" If you are still hungry after a careful re-evaluation, slide a little bit more food to the center of the plate. If you have finished all the food on your plate and are still hungry, add more to your plate but follow the same procedure of creating central and outside regions. The idea is to continually set up visible regions to give yourself an idea of how much food you really need.[31]

You have committed yourself to losing weight with the Medifast Program, you have set realistic weight-loss goals, and you have learned key elements of behavior change. Now that you are in the right mind-set and are equipped with the necessary tools for successful weight loss, it is time to learn about the Medifast 5 & 1 Plan.

Debbie Dewey

lost 61 pounds with Medifast

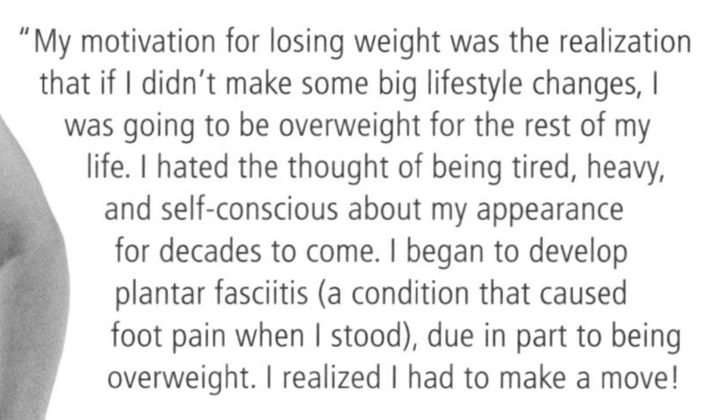

"My motivation for losing weight was the realization that if I didn't make some big lifestyle changes, I was going to be overweight for the rest of my life. I hated the thought of being tired, heavy, and self-conscious about my appearance for decades to come. I began to develop plantar fasciitis (a condition that caused foot pain when I stood), due in part to being overweight. I realized I had to make a move!

"I tried other weight-loss programs, but did not have much success. I lost weight, but immediately gained it all back, plus more. A friend of mine was successful with Medifast, so I figured if she could do it, then so could I. Once I started Medifast, I noticed results almost immediately! I started losing weight within days, and after my first two weeks, I was already feeling better physically.

"On Medifast, all of the work was done for me: The correct balance of vitamins, calories, protein, fat, and carbohydrates was provided in each Medifast Meal. All I had to do was follow the program, and I lost the weight—it was very simple!

"I now feel twenty years younger! I can now shop in the petite clothing department, tuck in a shirt, wear a belt, and run three miles—thanks, Medifast!"

Results will vary. This success story lost weight using a Medifast Weight Control Center Program.

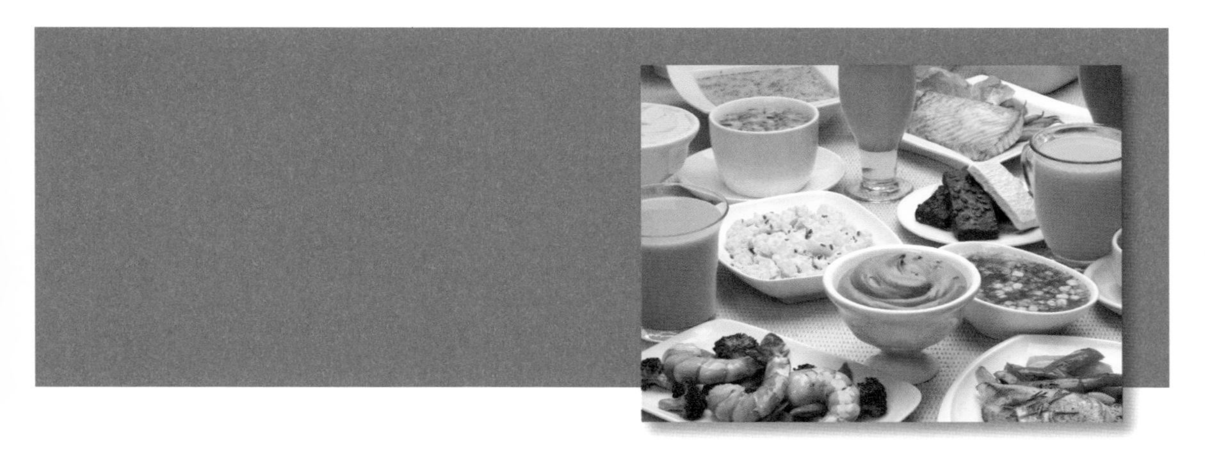

6 The Medifast 5 & 1 Plan

Before you get started on the Medifast Program, you will want to spend some time planning and organizing. Remember to identify the reasons you wish to lose weight. Determine what your goals will be. Familiarize yourself with potential roadblocks to your weight-loss success. Pre-plan how you are going to deal with the roadblocks. Have your support network in place. Make sure the timing is right.

Let's get started

Step one: See your doctor

Before you begin the Medifast 5 & 1 Plan (or any diet), you may want to schedule an appointment with your physician or qualified medical practitioner for a check-up, especially if you: are over the age of 70, have diabetes (or any other serious medical conditions), have 50 or more pounds to lose; or are taking medications. Some tests to ask about include complete blood count (CBC), complete metabolic/chemistry panel, lipid profile, thyroid panel, urinalysis, and electrocardiogram (ECG).

Step two: Gather your supplies

You'll want to order at least a 2-week supply (and ideally a 4-week supply) of Medifast Meals before you start, and continue ordering on a monthly schedule. Schedule your reorders in advance so you don't run out of your meals.

Before you start, you'll need:

- At-least a 2-week supply of Medifast Meals (ideally a 4-week supply)
- A shaker jar (free with your first order) or blender
- Snack products
- A journal or notebook to record your progress

Step three: Start your Plan

The Medifast 5 & 1 Plan was medically designed to create a calorie deficit, allowing your body to burn fat for energy. Each nutritionally balanced Medifast Meal is formulated with a proven combination of carbohydrates and protein, allowing you to successfully lose weight while maintaining lean muscle mass. The 5 & 1 Plan provides between 800 and 1,000 calories per day from 5 portion-controlled, nutritionally balanced Medifast Meals, plus 1 Lean & Green Meal.

Because Medifast is a low-calorie, low-fat, and moderately low-carbohydrate plan, it is a proportionately higher protein weight-loss plan. The latest research from the OmniHeart (Optimal Macronutrient Intake Trial to Prevent Heart Disease) diet study shows that a diet plan containing a lower proportion of carbohydrates and a higher proportion of protein has the best health benefits in terms of reducing blood pressure and LDL (bad) cholesterol levels.[32]

Because Medifast is low in both calories and carbohydrates, your body is forced to look elsewhere for energy. Initially, the carbohydrates your body stores as glycogen in the liver and muscles will provide you with fuel to run on. But after about two or three days on the Medifast Program, these stores will be used up and your body will start metabolizing fat stores for energy. Your body will not use up as much protein stores (a major component of muscle mass) because Medifast's nutritional formula maintains a consistent level of protein in your bloodstream, which protects muscle tissue from being burned for energy.

On the Medifast 5 & 1 Plan, your body enters a fat-burning state. The fat-burning state is a normal adaptive mechanism that your body uses to manage energy. The nutrient balance of Medifast (in combination with the low calorie level) causes the body's fat stores to release free fatty acids, which are then converted by the liver into an energy source called ketones. The fat-burning state achieved on the Medifast 5 & 1 Plan is very mild, and helps the body achieve rapid weight loss while preserving muscle tissue. The fat-burning state also helps eliminate hunger while providing sufficient levels of energy. It generally takes about three to five days to get into the fat-burning state. The best way to determine if you are in the fat-burning state is by recognizing physical clues—such as feeling less hungry and more energized.

The Medifast 5 & 1 Plan

Now that you understand how Medifast helps you lose weight, you may begin your weight-loss plan. Everyday, is as simple as:

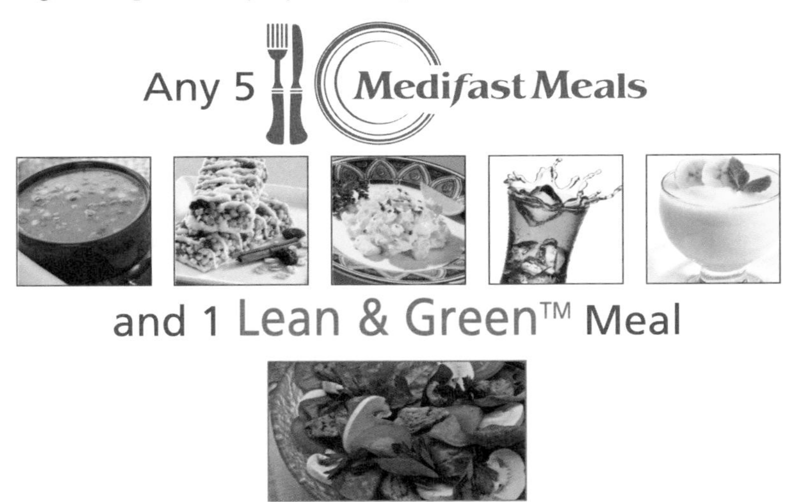

By having six meals a day (5 Medifast Meals and 1 Lean & Green Meal) you can lose weight steadily and safely. There are over 70 Medifast Meals to choose from. Remember, you may choose any combination of Meals on your 5 & 1 Plan including shakes, soups, oatmeal, puddings and more!

What should my Lean & Green Meal look like?

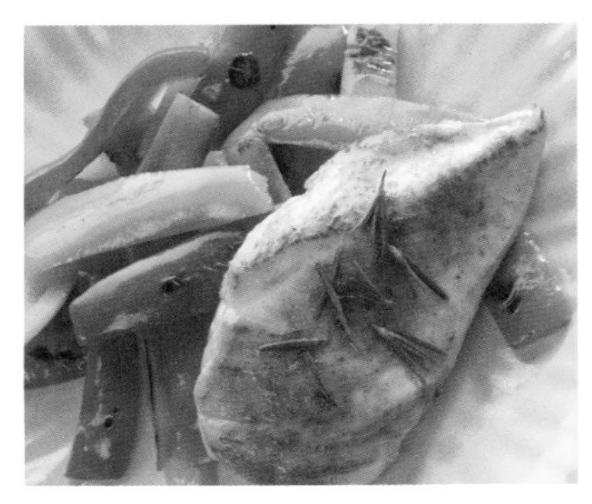

Your Lean & Green Meal should include a balance of lean protein and salad or vegetables. Choose five to seven ounces of lean protein (e.g., chicken, fish, tofu), and three servings of vegetables (raw or cooked, your choice). The combination of the fiber (from the veggies) and the protein will help to keep you feeling full longer.

Tips for success

The first few days

Achieving the fat-burning state on the Medifast 5 & 1 Plan takes two to five days. During this time you may feel tired, hungry, or irritable as your body adjusts.

This is temporary, so hang in there. Within about 72 hours you start to burn fat, and you'll feel energized and less hungry—and you'll get the thrill of seeing success. Here are some tips to get you through the first few days:

- If you're really struggling with hunger or fatigue in your first days, don't give up, have an extra Medifast Shake. It's better to have an extra Shake than to go off your program. Remind yourself you are on a journey to improve your health and take it one step at a time.
- Stay busy and occupied.
- Avoid tempting sights and smells of foods until you feel strong enough to resist overeating. Do whatever it takes.
- Log onto MyMedifast.com and chat with other newcomers—as well as more long-term customers—who can offer support and encouragement.

Space your meals carefully

Start each day with a schedule, and know the specific times you will eat your meals. Build six time slots for meals into your daily routine, keeping the times as consistent as possible. On weekends, your schedule might change a little, so shift your meal times accordingly.

Otherwise plan to have your Medifast Meals every two to three hours. Have your first one soon after you get up in the morning. If you can't eat that early, plan to have your shake or bar as soon as you get to work. Unless your schedule requires that you sleep late, have your first meal before 9:00 a.m. to allow adequate spacing and to minimize the feeling of hunger. Studies show that many overweight people skip breakfast. Skipping breakfast is a setup for failure. Breakfast helps to prevent hunger later on. Hunger is an unwanted temptation that can lead to a food binge.

Use Medifast Meals at meal times that cause you the most trouble. For instance, if breakfast is always an on-the-run donut, then drink a Medifast Shake instead. If you routinely skip lunch, or succumb to fast-food advertisements, grab a Medifast Bar instead. If you can't find the time to make a healthy dinner, but breakfast is easy, then have your Lean & Green Meal in the morning and a Medifast Meal for dinner. There is no rule that your Lean & Green Meal must be at dinnertime.

If you work evening or night hours, schedule your meals based on when your day begins. For example if you start your day at 4:00 p.m., plan out your meal times for the hours you are normally awake. Have your first meal when you wake up, and then keep your remaining meals spaced two to three hours apart.

Don't skip meals

Eating consistently will ensure quick, steady weight loss, so make sure you eat all five Medifast Meals and one Lean & Green Meal in a 24-hour period. Another reason to get in all your meals is because Medifast Meals contain the minimum amount of nutrients required by your body, so missing any of them will drop you below the minimum level. Remember that your body is a finely-tuned machine that can't run on empty.

Because you don't feel hungry you may be tempted to skip a meal. Don't! Not feeling very hungry is one of the nicest benefits of Medifast. But to maintain that benefit, you have to eat your meals consistently. Skipping meals because you're not hungry will throw you off balance. Your body will protect itself by conserving calories and slowing your metabolism. The bottom line is that skipping meals may actually slow your weight loss!

Eat slowly

Spend at least 10 to 15 minutes eating a Medifast Meal. Use a straw for shakes and drinks. Cut bars into small pieces to help you slow down while eating. Remember to savor your foods by eating them mindfully. Chew each bite of food at least 20 times before swallowing.

Drink lots of fluids

During weight loss, your body will require extra fluids to eliminate the by-products of fat metabolism. Water doesn't cause you to lose weight, but it increases your body's efficiency by eliminating the body's toxins and will help your scale show the consistent result you're looking for.

During your program, drink at least eight glasses (64 ounces) of water or other non-caloric beverages a day. If you have trouble getting this much in, then start with three to four glasses a day and gradually increase. Low-calorie and non-caloric beverages include unsweetened hot or iced tea, herbal tea, coffee, diet sodas, sparkling water, and sugar-free drink mixes.

Limit caffeine

It is best to limit coffee and caffeinated drinks to three servings a day. The low-calorie level of Medifast Meals may increase your sensitivity to caffeine, which may cause anxiety, shakiness, or other symptoms.

Avoid alcohol

Alcoholic beverages—even low-carb versions—are not recommended on the Medifast Program. Alcohol provides unneeded calories and even one drink can slow your weight loss. Alcohol provides extra calories with no nutritional value, stimulates the appetite (encouraging additional food intake), and can deplete your body of needed water.

Watch out for additional calories and carbohydrates

Just one slice of bread or piece of cake can put you out of the fat-burning state. If your weight loss slows down, you may be eating off the plan, even if you are not aware. Just small amounts of high-carbohydrate or high-calorie food can really add up.

Snacks you may have

Look for ways to protect yourself from the wrong foods. As much as possible, stay away from food until you feel strong enough to resist temptations. The weight loss you achieve during the first week on Medifast will help keep you going!

If you really must chew on something, grab three stalks of celery. Celery has a high water content and contains minimal calories. You may also chew sugar free gum and mints, but limit to five pieces per day because these products can contain carbohydrates. One cup of bouillon, two pickle spears, or one-half cup of sugar-free Jello®, are also acceptable snacks. Snacks are optional. If you choose to include a snack, please limit to one per day.

Be creative

Many people use our shaker jars for their Medifast drinks. If you like your drinks extra cold, add some ice cubes or crushed ice to the water. Some people use blenders, then add the ice and the packets together. This makes a filling smoothie drink. To vary the texture, try playing with the amounts of water and ice.

Some people choose to use fancy glasses and goblets, others choose to relax with a favorite mug. Find what works best for you. But drink your shake mindfully. This is your meal and you'll want to enjoy it. Avoid drinking standing up or on the go, so you feel like you're getting the full meal experience.

Medifast foods come in a wide range of types and flavors. In addition to the shakes, you can have hot soups, cocoa, teas, scrambled eggs, beef stew, oatmeal, chili, bars and more! Mix and match so you don't get bored. For example, have Medifast Oatmeal for breakfast, a Shake mid-morning, a Bar for lunch, a Shake late afternoon, your Lean & Green Meal for dinner, and Pudding for dessert in the evening.

Reaching your goal

You may stay on the 5 & 1 Plan until you have lost your desired amount of weight. Making positive lifestyle changes takes time and practice. Don't get discouraged if you are not perfect and fall off plan. One day is never enough to stop you from losing. Even if you feel you have slowed your weight-loss progress, get back on track as quickly as possible. If you have eaten food that is not on the 5 & 1 Plan, have a Medifast Meal and continue where you left off—ensuring that you get in all 5 Medifast Meals that day. Learn from your experiences and get back on track as quickly as possible. If you do get out of the fat-burning state, continue with your 5 Medifast Meals and 1 Lean & Green Meal—and within three days you will be back on track. Don't give up.

After you have reached your goal weight, you will need to transition into the weight-maintenance phase. This part of the Medifast Program is an absolute necessity so that you don't regain any of the weight you just lost. You didn't just do all this hard work for nothing! Chapter 7 will show you everything you need to know about Transition and Maintenance, and how to continue your healthy new lifestyle with Medifast.

10 Reasons Why I Want To Maintain My Weight Loss

1. ______________________________

2. ______________________________

3. ______________________________

4. ______________________________

5. ______________________________

6. ______________________________

7. ______________________________

8. ______________________________

9. ______________________________

10. ______________________________

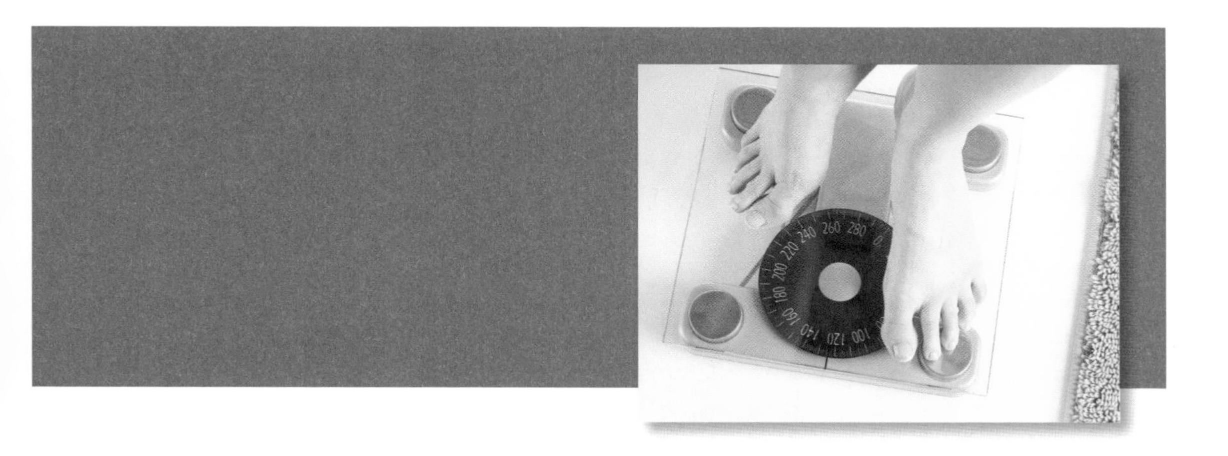

7 Transition and Maintenance

Congratulations, you have worked very hard to reach your goal weight! As you begin to transition into the weight-maintenance phase, it is important to recall the reasons why you wanted to lose weight in the first place. In chapter 6 you were asked to write down 10 reasons for wanting to reach your goal weight. Now, please write down 10 reasons why you want to keep your weight off. Make sure these are personal reasons, not what you think others want. Any time you need reinforcement, refer to this list.

Transition Plan

Upon reaching your goal weight, you will then transition from the Medifast 5 & 1 Plan into a phase we call Maintenance. Transition and Maintenance provide the keys to maintaining your weight-loss results on a long-term basis. During Transition and Maintenance, you will be reintroduced to foods you previously put on hold—foods such as fruits, low-fat dairy products, whole grains, and higher-carbohydrate vegetables.

Remember, Medifast is a lifestyle change, not just a short term weight-loss solution. Healthy eating provides the foundation for your new, healthy lifestyle.

Don't worry if you experience some weight fluctuation at the start of

Transition—this is perfectly normal! As you move out of the fat-burning state, your fluid levels may shift, which may cause a few pounds weight fluctuation. These changes are temporary, and over time, your weight should remain consistent.

During Transition, you incrementally increase your daily caloric intake by reintroducing a different food group each week. The Transition Plan isn't one-size-fits-all. Your gender, age, height, weight, and activity level will determine your calorie requirements. In order to help pinpoint a calorie level appropriate for you, please refer to Calculating your basal metabolic rate (BMR).

The information provided below will give you an idea of how long you should remain in Transition—depending upon the amount of weight you lost:

- If you lost less than 50 pounds, allow 8 weeks to transition.
- If you lost 50 to 100 pounds, allow 12 weeks to transition.
- If you lost more than 100 pounds, allow 16 weeks to transition.

The first four weeks of Transition are similar for everyone. You'll incrementally increase your daily caloric intake with a different food group each week. This is done in weekly stages:

Stage 1: Additional vegetables

Stage 2: Fruits

Stage 3: Dairy

Stage 4: Whole grains

For your convenience, we've included sample Transition Plan charts. These sample charts are tailored to those looking to ultimately maintain their weight-loss results with a 1,500 per day meal plan.

Transition Plan chart

For weight loss of less than 50 pounds.

Stage	Plan
Stage 1: Additional vegetables Week 1 (900–1,050 calories) Any of your favorite vegetables can now be added back to your diet.	5 Medifast Meals 1 Lean & Green Meal **1 additional cup vegetables**
Stage 2: Fruits Week 2 (900–1,050 calories) Fresh fruit is desired but if canned fruit is used, choose unsweetened or packed in juice–not syrup.	4 Medifast Meals 1 Lean & Green Meal 1 additional cup vegetables **1 medium-sized piece of fruit or ½ cup cubed fruit or berries**
Stage 3: Dairy Week 3 (1,000–1,050 calories) Dairy includes low-fat and/or sugar-free yogurt, milk, or Lactaid® product.	4 Medifast Meals 1 Lean & Green Meal 1 additional cup vegetables 1 medium-sized piece of fruit or ½ cup cubed fruit or berries **½ cup low-fat or fat-free dairy**
Stage 4: Whole grains Week 4–8 (1,350–1,500 calories) Whole grain can be 1 slice of whole-grain bread, ½ whole-grain English muffin, ¾ cup high-fiber cereal, ½ cup whole-wheat pasta, or ½ cup brown rice.	3 Medifast Meals 1 Lean & Green Meal 1 additional cup vegetables, raw or cooked 2 medium-sized pieces of fruit or 1 cup of cubed fruit or berries 1 cup low-fat or fat-free diary **1 serving whole grain** **Additional 4-6 oz of meat, chicken, fish, or seafood that is baked, poached, or broiled–not fried**

Transition Plan chart

For weight loss of 50 to 100 pounds.

Stage	Daily plan
Stage 1: Additional vegetables Week 1 (900–1,050 calories) Any of your favorite vegetables can now be added back to your diet.	5 Medifast Meals 1 Lean & Green Meal **1 additional cup vegetables**
Stage 2: Fruits Week 2 (900–1,050 calories) Fresh fruit is desired but if canned fruit is used, choose unsweetened or packed in juice–not syrup.	4 Medifast Meals 1 Lean & Green Meal 1 additional cup vegetables **1 medium-sized piece of fruit or ½ cup cubed fruit or berries**
Stage 3: Dairy Week 3 (1,000–1,050 calories) Dairy includes low-fat and/or sugar-free yogurt, milk, or Lactaid® product.	4 Medifast Meals 1 Lean & Green Meal 1 additional cup vegetables 1 medium-sized piece of fruit or ½ cup cubed fruit or berries **½ cup low-fat or fat-free dairy**
Stage 4: Whole grains Week 4–12 (1,350–1,500 calories) Whole grain can be 1 slice of whole-grain bread, ½ whole-grain English muffin, ¾ cup high-fiber cereal, ½ cup whole-wheat pasta, or ½ cup brown rice.	3 Medifast Meals 1 Lean & Green Meal 1 additional cup vegetables, raw or cooked 2 medium-sized pieces of fruit or 1 cup of cubed fruit or berries 1 cup low-fat or fat-free diary **1 serving whole grain** **Additional 4-6 oz of meat, chicken, fish, or seafood that is baked, poached, or broiled–not fried**

Transition Plan chart

For weight loss of more than 100 pounds.

Stage	Daily plan
Stage 1: Additional vegetables Week 1 (900–1,050 calories) Any of your favorite vegetables can now be added back to your diet.	5 Medifast Meals 1 Lean & Green Meal **1 additional cup vegetables**
Stage 2: Fruits Week 2 (900–1,050 calories) Fresh fruit is desired but if canned fruit is used, choose unsweetened or packed in juice–not syrup.	4 Medifast Meals 1 Lean & Green Meal 1 additional cup vegetables **1 medium-sized piece of fruit or ½ cup cubed fruit or berries**
Stage 3: Dairy Week 3 (1,000–1,050 calories) Dairy includes low-fat and/or sugar-free yogurt, milk, or Lactaid® product.	4 Medifast Meals 1 Lean & Green Meal 1 additional cup vegetables 1 medium-sized piece of fruit or ½ cup cubed fruit or berries **½ cup low-fat or fat-free dairy**
Stage 4: Whole grains Week 4–16 (1,350–1,500 calories) Whole grain can be 1 slice of whole-grain bread, ½ whole-grain English muffin, ¾ cup high-fiber cereal, ½ cup whole-wheat pasta, or ½ cup brown rice.	3 Medifast Meals 1 Lean & Green Meal 1 additional cup vegetables, raw or cooked 2 medium-sized pieces of fruit or 1 cup of cubed fruit or berries 1 cup low-fat or fat-free diary **1 serving whole grain** **Additional 4-6 oz of meat, chicken, fish, or seafood that is baked, poached, or broiled–not fried**

Your ending calorie level during Transition is essentially your starting point for Maintenance. In Maintenance, you'll learn to sustain your weight-loss results by making healthy food choices and living an active lifestyle.

Maintenance

Maintenance essentially is the process of sustaining your weight-loss results by making healthy food choices and living an active lifestyle. You'll soon discover that Maintenance is a perpetual "calorie balancing and monitoring act." The ultimate goal of Maintenance is to help you remain at a healthy weight for the rest of your life.

During the weight-loss phase, your goal was to take in less energy (calories) than you were burning until you reached your goal weight. Now that you have reached your goal weight, you will want your energy intake to be more or less equal to the energy you burn. This is the point at which your body weight is in balance with your food intake and activity level.

For many individuals, Maintenance begins with a 1,500 calorie per day diet. However, the actual number of calories you need to maintain a stable weight over the long term is individual—and varies depending on factors such as gender, age, height, weight, and activity level. You may need to experiment with different calorie levels during Maintenance in order to find what level is right for you.

In order to help pinpoint a calorie level appropriate for your gender, age, height, and weight, please refer to Calculating Your Basal Metabolic Rate. This section will help you determine your Total Energy Expenditure (TEE). TEE is based upon your BMR, Thermic Effect of Food (TEF), and Physical Activity Level (PAL).

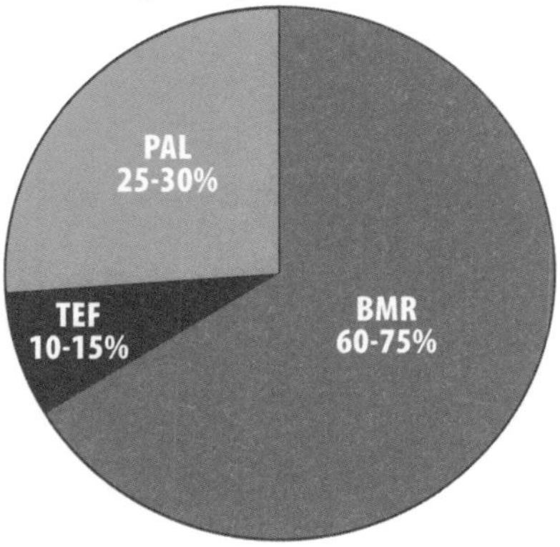

BMR refers to the amount of energy (calories) expended while at rest. TEF refers to the energy used to metabolize food and use it for fuel. PAL is the most variable piece of the equation and is based on how physically active you are. Determining your TEE (and sticking with a meal plan calorie level based around your TEE) greatly improves your chances of sustaining the weight-loss results you've worked so hard to achieve.

The 5 & 1 Plan helped you develop healthful eating habits. Eating small, frequent meals (six times per day) of portion-controlled, nutritious food is a great habit to carry over into Maintenance. Many customers who have worked hard to achieve a healthy weight, find success by continuing to eat two to three Medifast Meals each day. This is a convenient way to keep calorie levels within range, and also helps you stick with your 6-times-per-day meal schedule.

One of the most common reasons people gain weight back after dieting is that they see their diet as the beginning and the end of the weight control process. Don't allow yourself to get into that mind set. The idea of balancing your food intake with the calories you burn is the key to weight maintenance. Remember to make healthy food choices and live an active lifestyle. Don't slip back into your old habits! Remember you need to keep moving daily and get exercising.

The two TEE Charts can be used as a reference. One chart is based on a 5'4" female and the other is based on a 5'10" male. To more accurately determine your recommended Maintenance calorie level, use the equation below.

Calculating your basal metabolic rate

In order to determine your BMR, use the Mifflin-St. Jeor Equation. Predictive energy equations are used to provide an estimate of your BMR. Of the four most commonly used predictive energy equations, the Mifflin-St Jeor equations give the most reliable results. To determine your BMR, enter your weight in pounds and your height in inches.

Step 1

Men
10 x (weight x 0.455) + 6.25 x (height x 2.54) - 5 x (age) + 5 = BMR

Women
10 x (weight x 0.455) + 6.25 x (height x 2.54) - 5 x (age) - 161 = BMR

Step 2

To determine your total daily calorie needs, the BMR has to be multiplied by the appropriate activity factor, as follows:

After determining your BMR, multiply by your Physical Activity Factor. Be honest with yourself as to your true activity level as PAL varies significantly between people. The result is your TEE. Your TEE is your recommended Maintenance calorie level.

Activity Factors:

1.200	Sedentary
1.375	Light activity *(light exercise/sports 1-3 days/week)*
1.550	Active *(moderate exercise/sports 3-5 days/week)*

1.725	Very active *(hard exercise/sports 6-7 days/week)*
1.900	Extra active *(very hard exercise/sports + physical job or 2x/day training)*

Total Energy Expenditure (BMR x PAL) for 5'4" female:

Age	Weight	BMR	TEE (Sedentary)	TEE (Light activity)	TEE (Active)	TEE (Very active)
	110	1162	1394	1597	1800	2004
	120	1207	1448	1660	1871	2082
20	130	1253	1503	1722	1941	2161
	140	1298	1558	1785	2012	2239
	150	1344	1612	1847	2082	2318
	110	1065	1277	1464	1652	1836
	120	1110	1332	1526	1721	1915
30	130	1156	1387	1589	1791	1993
	140	1201	1441	1714	1932	2150
	150	1247	1496	1906	2149	2392
	110	968	1161	1330	1500	1669
	120	1013	1216	1393	1570	1747
40	130	1059	1270	1455	1641	1826
	140	1104	1325	1518	1711	1904
	150	1150	1379	1581	1782	1983
	110	871	1045	1197	1349	1502
	120	916	1099	1260	1420	1580
50	130	962	1154	1322	1490	1659
	140	1007	1208	1385	1561	1737
	150	1053	1263	1447	1631	1816
	110	774	928	1064	1199	1334
	120	819	983	1126	1269	1413
60	130	865	1037	1189	1340	1491
	140	910	1092	1251	1411	1570
	150	956	1147	1314	1481	1648
	110	677	812	930	1049	1167
	120	722	866	993	1119	1245
70	130	768	921	1055	1190	1324
	140	813	976	1118	1260	1402
	150	859	1030	1180	1331	1481

Total Energy Expenditure (BMR x PAL) for 5'10" male:

Age	Weight	BMR	TEE (Sedentary)	TEE (Light activity)	TEE (Active)	TEE (Very active)
20	150	1065	1926	2207	2487	2768
	160	1650	1980	2269	2558	2847
	170	1696	2035	2332	2628	2925
	180	1741	2090	2394	2699	3004
30	150	1508	1809	2073	2337	2601
	160	1553	1864	2136	2408	2679
	170	1599	1919	2198	2478	2758
	180	1644	1973	2261	2549	2836
40	150	1411	1693	1940	2187	2434
	160	1456	1748	2002	2257	2512
	170	1502	1802	2065	2328	2591
	180	1547	1857	2127	2398	2669
50	150	1314	1577	1806	2036	2266
	160	1359	1631	1869	2107	2345
	170	1405	1686	1932	2177	2423
	180	1450	1740	1994	2248	2502
60	150	1217	1460	1673	1886	2099
	160	1262	1515	1736	1956	2177
	170	1308	1569	1798	2027	2256
	180	1353	1624	1861	2098	2334
70	150	1120	1344	1540	1736	1932
	160	1165	1398	1602	1806	2010
	170	1211	1453	1665	1877	2089
	180	1256	1508	1727	1947	2167

Eating healthy

During Transition and Maintenance, you will once again be eating fruits, low-fat dairy products, whole grains, and higher-carbohydrate vegetables. The following information will help you select healthy foods—tips for what to eat, what to purchase, and what to be wary of in non-Medifast foods!

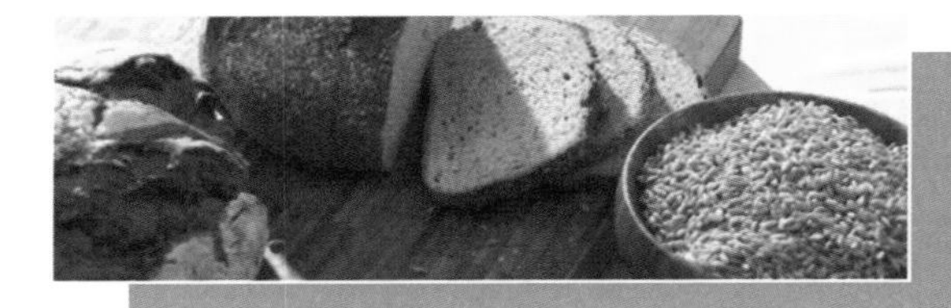

Grains

Examples of one grain serving:

- 1 cup unsweetened cereal
- ½ cup cooked cereal
- ⅓ cup cooked brown rice
- ½ cup cooked whole-wheat pasta
- 1 slice whole-grain bread

Choose these foods...	...instead of these foods
Whole-grain bread	Refined white bread
Brown rice	White rice
Whole-wheat pasta	Refined flour pasta
Whole-wheat flour	Refined flour
Whole-grain breakfast cereal	Sugary breakfast cereal

* Choose foods with whole oats, whole rye, or whole wheat listed first on the label's ingredients list.
* Look for breads with at least two grams of fiber per slice.
* Be wary of foods labeled multi-grain, stone ground, 100% wheat, or bran. These are usually NOT whole-grain products.
* Choose foods with fewer added sugars, fats, or oils.

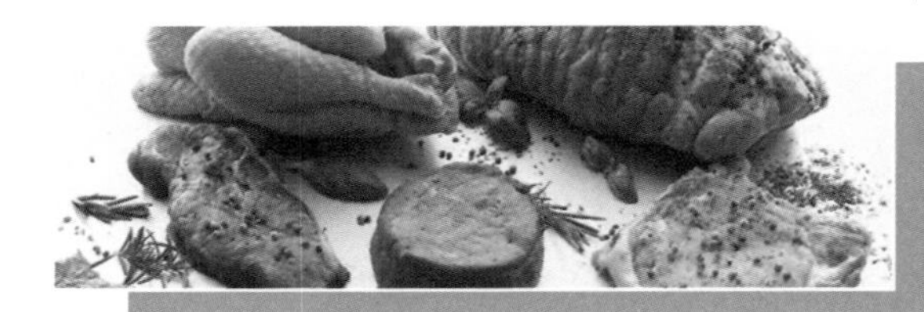

Protein

Examples of one serving of protein: four to six ounces (cooked weight) of any lean meat (or meat substitute):

- skinless chicken or turkey *(white meat preferred)*
- white fish *(fresh or frozen cod, flounder, haddock, halibut, trout)*, tuna *(fresh or canned in water)*, smoked salmon, salmon *(fresh or canned)*
- shellfish *(clams, crabs, lobster, scallops, shrimp, imitation shell fish)*
- duck, venison, buffalo, or ostrich
- egg whites or egg substitutes
- low-fat or fat-free cottage cheese
- low-fat or fat-free cheese
- processed sandwich meats with one gram of fat or less per oz *(such as deli-thin meats)*, including turkey, roast beef, and ham
- USDA Select or Choice grades of lean beef trimmed of fat: round, sirloin, and flank steak; tenderloin; roast *(rib, chuck, rump)*; steak *(T-bone, porterhouse)*, ground round
- lamb *(roast, chop, leg)*
- veal *(lean chop, roast)*
- ½ cup beans or lentils *(cooked)*

Choose these foods...	...instead of these foods
Boneless, skinless chicken breast	Chicken thighs with skin
Lean ground beef (85-99% lean)	Regular ground beef (70-84% lean)
Grilled, baked, or broiled meats	Deep-fried meats

* Choose lean cuts of beef and pork such as loin and round cuts.
* Choose skinless poultry. Bake, broil, poach, or grill—do not fry.
* Each week, eat at least two servings of fish rich in omega-3 fatty acids, including salmon, albacore tuna, mackerel, trout, or herring.
* Choose meat substitutes made with soybeans or textured vegetable protein, legume-type beans, egg whites, egg substitutes, or low-fat cheeses.

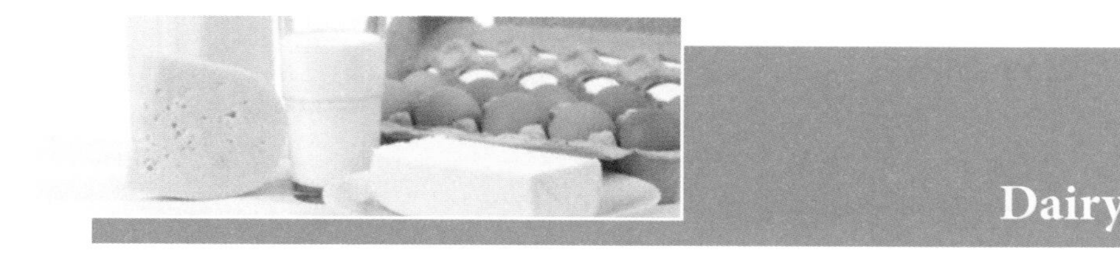

Dairy

Examples of one dairy serving:

- 1 cup skim or 1% low-fat milk
- 1 cup low-fat or fat-free milk or soy milk

- 1 cup low-fat or fat-free buttermilk
- ½ cup fat free evaporated milk
- 1 cup fat-free non-nutritive sweetened and/or fructose-sweetened yogurt
- ½ cup fat-free or low-fat yogurt

Choose these foods...	...instead of these foods
Skim or 1% milk	2% milk/whole milk
Fat-free/low-fat yogurt	Whole-milk yogurt

* Always choose fat-free or low-fat milk, cheese, and yogurt. Cheese can also be used as a substitute for lean meat.
* Sweetened milk products such as condensed milk or flavored milk contain added sugars (which increase calories), so be careful when consuming.
* Choose sugar-free yogurt.

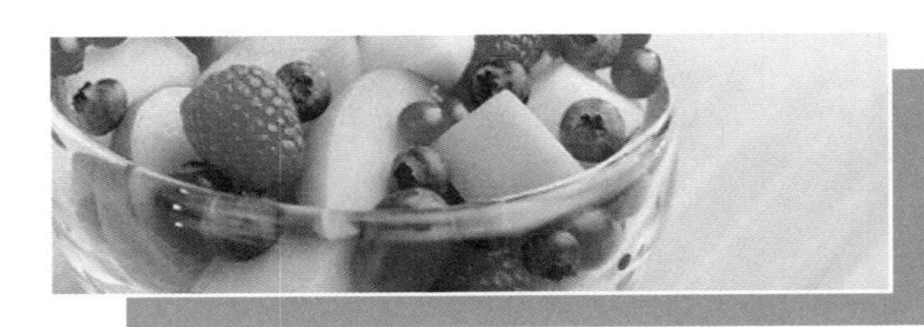

Fruits and vegetables

- Strive for at least two servings of fruit per day (one serving = one medium-sized piece of fruit or ½ cup of cubed fruit or berries) and three servings of vegetables per day (one serving = ½ cup cooked vegetable or 1 cup raw).
- Choose fresh, frozen, or canned fruits or vegetables without added fat or sauce.
- Add vegetables back into your program—even the ones that are higher in carbohydrates such as corn, peas, and potatoes. All vegetables are healthy, provide fiber to help fill you up, are low in calories, and are packed with vitamins and minerals.

* Choose **BLUE/PURPLE** from eggplant, blueberries, or blackberries to help maintain: a lower risk of some cancers; urinary tract health; memory funcion; healthy aging.*
* Add **GREEN** from broccoli, peas, celery, cabbage, grapes, limes, pears or kiwi

fruit to your diet to maintain: a lower risk of some cancers; vision health; strong bones and teeth.*

* Working **WHITE** from cauliflower, garlic, mushrooms, onions, white corn, bananas, or white peaches into your diet helps maintain: heart health; cholesterol levels that are already healthy; a lower risk of some cancers.*
* Make **YELLOW/ORANGE** from carrots, yellow squash, pumpkin, sweet potatoes, apricots, mango, pineapple, lemons, or oranges as part of your diet to help maintain: heart health; vision health; a healthy immune system; a lower risk of some cancers.*
* Be sure to include **RED** from beets, radishes, tomatoes, apples, strawberries, raspberries, cherries, or watermelon in your low-fat diet to help maintain: heart health; memory function; a lower risk of some cancers; urinary tract health.*

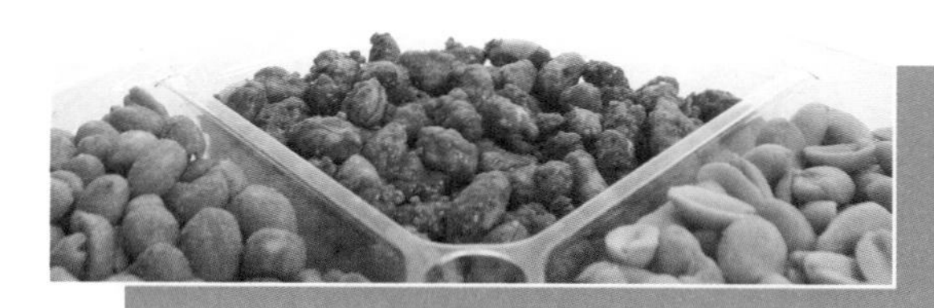

Fats and other foods

Examples of one fat serving:

Monounsaturated	Polyunsaturated	Saturated
• 1 tsp olive or canola oil	• 2 Tbsp low-fat dressing	• 1 tsp butter
• 8 large black olives	• 1 tsp mayonnaise	• 2 Tbsp cream or half and half
• 10 large pimento-stuffed green olives	• 1 Tbsp reduced-fat mayonnaise	• 1 Tbsp cream cheese
• ½ Tbsp peanut butter	• 2 walnuts	• 2 Tbsp sour cream
• 6 almonds or mixed nuts	• 2 tsp Miracle Whip® salad dressing	• 3 Tbsp reduced-fat cream cheese
• 10 peanuts	• 1 Tbsp reduced-fat Miracle Whip®	• 1 slice bacon
• 1 Tbsp sesame seeds	• 1 Tbsp pumpkin seeds or sunflower seeds	
• ⅛ avocado	• 1 tsp trans fat-free margarine	

*Diets rich in fruits and vegetables may reduce the risk of some types of cancer and other chronic diseases.

Choose these foods...	...instead of these foods
Margarine that is free of trans fats	Butter
Small amounts of nuts and seeds	Chocolate and high-calorie desserts
Calorie-free beverages	Sugary drinks
Oils high in omega-3 such as canola, soybean, peanut, or olive oil	Palm, palm kernel, or coconut oil

* Choose mostly monounsaturated fats, moderate amounts of polyunsaturated fats, and less saturated fats for improved heart health.

The tables below can help you find a Maintenance meal plan appropriate for your calorie needs. It is designed to help you make wise food choices in accordance with your desired calorie level. Please refer to the back of the book for sample meal plans based upon a 1,500 calorie per day intake.

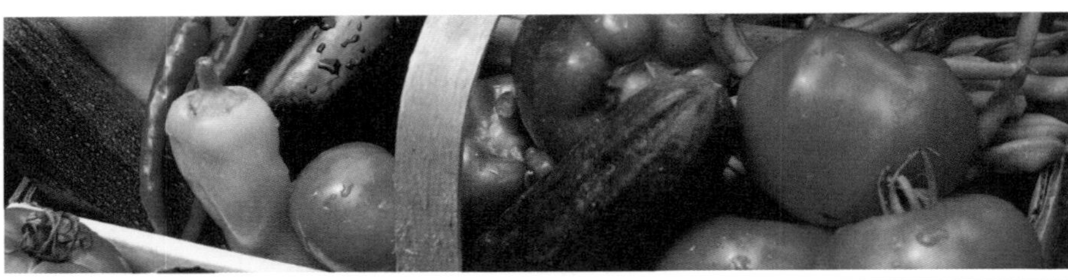

Servings based on your estimated daily caloric goal (BMR x PAL). Servings are listed as a number to have each day.	**1,200 calories**	**1,500 calories**	**1,800 calories**	**2,000 calories**
Medifast Meals	2	3	3	3
Grain serving	1	1	2	2
Vegetable serving	3	3	3	3
Fruit serving	1	2	2	3
Protein serving	2 4-oz servings	2 4-oz servings	2 4- to 6-oz servings	2 6-oz servings
Dairy serving	2	2	3	3
Fat serving	1	2	3	4

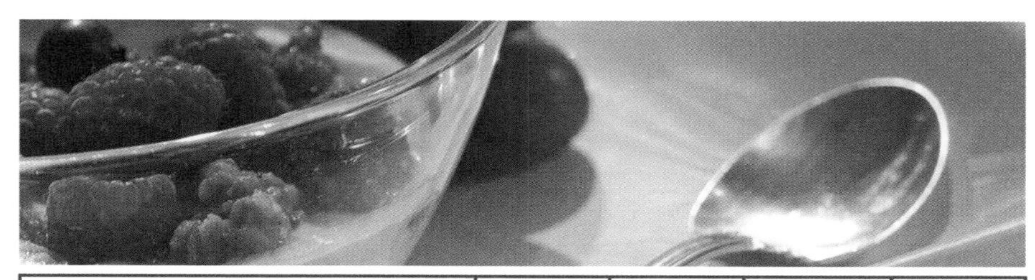

Servings based on your estimated daily caloric goal (BMR x PAL). Servings are listed as a number to have each day.	2,200 calories	2,400 calories	2,500 calories	2,600 calories
Medifast Meals	3	4	4	4
Grain serving	3	4	4	6
Vegetable serving	4	4	4	4
Fruit serving	4	4	4	4
Protein serving	2 6-oz servings	2 6-oz servings	2 6-oz servings	2 7-oz servings
Dairy serving	3	3	4	4
Fat serving	5	5	5	5

Servings based on your estimated daily caloric goal (BMR x PAL). Servings are listed as a number to have each day.	2,700 calories	2,800 calories	2,900 calories	3,000 calories
Medifast Meals	4	5	5	5
Grain serving	7	7	8	9
Vegetable serving	4	4	4	4
Fruit serving	4	4	4	4
Protein serving	2 7-oz servings	2 7-oz servings	2 7-oz servings	2 7-oz servings
Dairy serving	4	4	4	4
Fat serving	5	5	6	6

Monitor, monitor, monitor!

IMPORTANT! Set up a regular schedule to monitor your weight and measurements. Many people do best by weighing themselves just once or twice a week. If possible, always weigh yourself the same time each day while wearing little or no clothing. Keep in mind that most people tend to weigh less in the early morning than late afternoon or evening. Monitoring your weight and measurements will soon become second nature.

Consider the scale (to monitor weight) and tape measure (to monitor inches) to be necessary tools of your new trade! Another excellent tip is to use a pair of jeans or your favorite pair of pants as a barometer. You know how they're supposed to fit. A tighter fit indicates that you may be putting on weight.

Determine a weight range that you plan to maintain over the course of time. Whenever the scale indicates you are at the upper limit of your weight range, consider it a red flag—and immediately assess what's going on in your life. Evaluate where you need to make changes and put them into action. Change any negative patterns now, rather than letting them spiral out of control.

The Medifast blitz

Should you reach or exceed the upper limit of your weight range, consider going back on the 5 & 1 Plan for a few weeks or just substitute one regular meal each day for a Medifast Meal until your weight comes back to a comfortable range. Take time to address any life issues that may be contributing to your weight gain:

- Have you let your exercise program slip?
- Are you allowing stress or other emotional issues affect your eating patterns?
- Are your portions too big?
- Are you eating too many meals away from home?

Take a careful look at where you might be slipping and change those patterns immediately. The Medifast Blitz can help you get back on track.

Plan for success

People often stray off course due to lack of planning. Remember the old adage,

"If you fail to plan, you plan to fail?" This certainly applies to Transition and Maintenance. Your odds for maintaining long-term weight-loss results greatly increase by creating (and sticking to) a realistic, individualized plan.

Doesn't your day seem to flow more smoothly when everything is organized on your calendar or within your planner? Success with Maintenance requires this type of organizational process—the more you plan ahead, the easier it will be to maintain your weight-loss results. Keep the following in mind:

Ask why. Why do you reach for extra food? Is it boredom? Stress? Peer pressure? Habit? Reward? Identify the reasons—then change the behavior.

Set goals. Your goals are commitments you make to yourself. Goals provide motivation for maintaining your weight loss.

Cooking fun. Many people view cooking as a chore. Cooking can be fun if you prepare and plan ahead. Plan dinners at the beginning of the week. Cut out new recipes, or ask your fellow Medifast friends about their favorite recipes. You can cook, pre-portion, and freeze in microwavable containers until ready to eat—for those meals on the run.

Schedule exercise. Scheduling exercise will make it a priority. Mark it on the calendar and make a date with yourself that cannot be broken. Also, track your exercise and see how it affects the scale.

Track your success. Since you've gotten used to tracking your weight loss, go ahead track other little successes, too like running with your kids, taking the stairs instead of the elevator, walking to the store instead of driving, or even walking your dog! These little activities are actually huge successes. Tracking them provides motivation—and serves to positively reinforce any increase in your daily activity level.

Portion control

Did you know that restaurant portions are now two to four times the size of standard serving sizes? Eating portion-controlled meals effectively reduces total calorie intake—and helps maintain weight-loss results.

Take note of serving sizes on product packages. Consider, for example, a 200-calorie, 20-ounce bottle of non-diet soda that lists 2.5 servings on the package. Since the calories listed on the package are per serving, you will have consumed 500 total calories by drinking the whole bottle.

Be mindful of portion sizes to help prevent overeating. Also be mindful to notice the flavors and textures of the foods you eat. Enjoy your food, and be thoughtful of every bite you put into your mouth. Try not to eat while performing other activities such as driving a car or watching television. Here are some easy visuals to help with portion sizes:

- 1 medium-sized fruit = ***size of a tennis ball***
- 1 cup of salad greens = ***size of a baseball***
- 1 ounce of cheese = ***size of a pair of dice***
- 4 ounces of cooked meat or chicken = ***size of a deck of playing cards or computer mouse***
- 1 teaspoon of butter or margarine = ***size of a fingertip***

Drink water

Water intake is an important part of the 5 & 1 Plan. It is equally important during Transition and Maintenance. Water does not cause you to lose weight, but it increases your body's efficiency by eliminating toxins. Water helps maintain muscle tone, promote weight loss, and develop healthy skin. It also helps prevent headaches, muscle and joint pain, bloating, and constipation. Drink at least eight glasses (64 ounces) of water a day.

In addition to the recommended 64-ounces of water per day, you can drink any liquids that are calorie-free. This includes unsweetened hot or iced tea, coffee, diet sodas, or other calorie-free beverages. You may use skim milk or fat-free half-and-half in your coffee or tea. You may also use artificial sweeteners, if desired.

Support helps

Studies have shown that for some individuals, peer support in combination with other weight maintenance strategies significantly improves the chances for maintaining weight-loss results. Peer support can be provided by family members and friends, or by coworkers and business associates, or weight-management groups. Your support system should offer advice and provide you with direction during difficult times. Your supportive friends and family can monitor your weight, encourage your progress, and praise your accomplishments.

While many people currently have a strong base of social support, others may find it more difficult to locate appropriate sources of help.

Helpful hints

Sustaining your weight-loss results requires dedication and determination. Maintenance becomes much easier when you embrace healthy eating and regular exercise. Learn how to cope with the ups and downs of everyday life, so you don't automatically reach for food during emotional or stressful times. Here are some helpful hints that can guide you through Transition and Maintenance:

Eat breakfast every day. High quality foods, such as Medifast Scrambled Eggs, Medifast Oatmeal, Medifast Cappuccino, or Medifast Chai Latte, are good choices to start your day right. You can also choose cooked oatmeal, an egg substitute, or high-fiber breakfast cereal. Research demonstrates that those who eat breakfast daily are most successful at maintaining a healthy weight.

Exercise daily. Exercise helps increase metabolism, strength, and flexibility. It also helps reduce stress and/or depression, and provides mental clarity. Those who can create a daily habit of exercise are most successful with maintaining their weight. Every activity counts!

Find support. Many people prefer to have support groups for motivation and guidance. Medifast offers support channels for everyone.

Eat low-fat meals six times a day. Eating six small meals per day controls portions and total caloric intake (especially those from fat). A meal can be a Medifast Meal, ½ a sandwich, or low-fat yogurt in between your larger meal periods.

Create an individual plan. Your odds for maintaining long-term weight-loss results greatly increase by creating (and sticking to) a realistic, individualized plan.

Monitor. Weigh yourself on a regular basis and strive to keep within your goal weight range. Those who monitor consistently are most successful at maintaining their weight.

Avoid trigger foods. You know the foods you always reach for during stressful situations? Get rid of them! If you know that strawberry ice cream is your downfall, don't buy it. If you have the urge to splurge, do an alternate activity for 10 minutes. This usually suppresses the urge. If it still persists, eat a very small portion to satisfy the craving.

Eat slowly. Spend at least 10 to 15 minutes eating your meals. Remember to savor your foods by eating them mindfully. Notice the taste and texture of the food. Chew each bite of food at least 20 times before swallowing.

Keep fresh vegetables in your refrigerator. If you pick at anything in the fridge, make it vegetables! Wash them, cut them, and leave them in the fridge for times you crave something to crunch on. Carrots and celery sticks are great for munching.

Take time to prepare foods. Tender loving preparation of food will be well worth your time. Prepared meals are healthier, taste better, and are more satisfying to eat.

Finding out about dining out

Going to restaurants can be Transition- and Maintenance-friendly! The following details what to look for, and what to watch out for.

Choose foods prepared this way:*

- Steamed
- Poached or broiled
- Baked
- Broiled or charbroiled
- Grilled or roasted
- Garden fresh

Avoid foods prepared this way:

- Fried, french fried, deep fried, batter fried, pan fried, or crispy
- Marinated in oil or butter, buttered, or buttery
- Creamed, creamy, cream sauce, or in its own gravy
- Au gratin or in cheese sauce
- Scampi style or breaded
- Scalloped or escalloped
- Pastry, rich, or a lá mode
- Peanut sauce or coconut milk

*Note: Items prepared by these methods are not necessarily low in fat since other fats may be added in the process (e.g., grilled items are usually brushed with oil before grilling; poached items may have butter added to the broth or inside the parchment pocket; baked items may have fats such as oil or cheese added; and marinara sauces often start with a base of oil). Also, if the cut of meat/fish/poultry used is high in fat, even with these cooking methods the food will likely still be high in fat. However, compared to items prepared by the methods in the *Avoid* section, these are likely to be relatively lower in fat.

Restaurant portion control tips

- Split your meal with somebody else in your group, or ask to be served a half-portion.
- Ask if the chef will put half the meal on your plate and half the meal in a doggie bag—they can keep the doggie bag in the kitchen until you're ready to go!

Ted Hasse

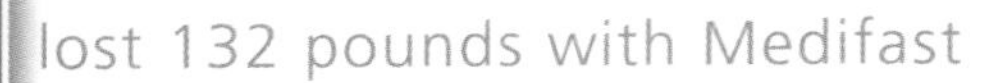

lost 132 pounds with Medifast

"I started the 5 & 1 Plan after a period of declining health. I woke up one night unable to breathe and was rushed to the emergency room. I was sent to numerous doctors who all said I was obese and needed to lose weight before I had a stroke, heart attack, or full-blown diabetes."

"I felt tired all the time and couldn't do the things my kids wanted me to do with them. I was embarrassed to be seen in a swimsuit, so I didn't go swimming on family vacations.

"My wife found out from a friend about the Medifast Program and she helped me to start! I noticed results within the first three or four days! I feel better now than I ever have. I have increased physical stamina and endurance, and I love to exercise now. My previous obesity-related medical conditions are non-existent. I feel almost 20 years younger!"

Results will vary.

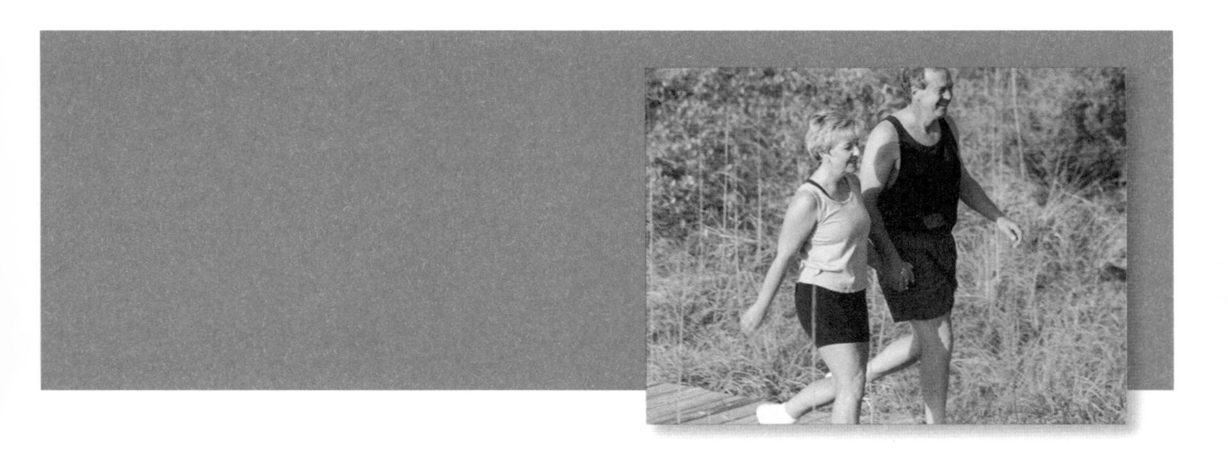

8 Get moving with Medifast

Move your body

Eating healthy is just the beginning of a healthy lifestyle. Exercise is also essential, and its benefits on your total well-being are enormous—it can even reduce your need for medications. A wealth of research studies confirms the role of exercise in weight loss and, particularly, in weight maintenance.

There are three basic types of exercise, and each of them can help with your weight-loss and weight-maintenance plans:

- Cardiovascular (aerobic) exercise burns calories. The longer and more intensely you exercise, the more calories you burn.
- Strength training increases lean muscle mass, which burns more calories than fat tissue. Having more muscle increases your metabolism, allowing you to burn more calories, even at rest, throughout the day.
- Lifestyle exercise can add to your daily calorie burn as well.

Energy balance

A "calorie" is a unit of measure used to express energy consumed and used by the body. The body gets calories through eating food, and burns calories through working and moving. Energy balance is the theory that your body's weight will remain the same when calories consumed are equal to calories expended. The Maintenance phase of the Medifast Program focuses on establishing and maintaining this balance.

When this balance is off, a person will gain or lose weight. It's quite simple, really: Weight gain results when you eat more calories than your body expends, either through eating too much food or moving the body too little—or both. Some medications such as corticosteroids, psychiatric medications, tranquilizers, select antidepressants, and medicines that increase fluid retention can also contribute to weight gain. Medical conditions such as Cushing's syndrome, untreated hypothyroidism, and polycystic ovary syndrome can also add pounds.

Weight loss results from a caloric deficit—when fewer calories are consumed than expended. You can create a caloric deficit in one of three ways:

- Eat fewer calories per day.
- Burn more calories with exercise.
- Eat less and burn more calories through exercise.

The Medifast Program advocates the third option for creating a healthy caloric deficit during the weight-loss phase of the program. The 5 & 1 Plan creates a caloric deficit with a calorie-controlled meal plan, and Medifast recommends incorporating an exercise program into your daily routine to help you burn calories and reap the additional health benefits of being active.

Although creating a caloric deficit is a good thing when it comes to the weight-loss phase, too much of a good thing can work against you. Too large of a calorie deficit can cause the body to conserve its energy stores, and actually slow down your weight loss. That's why it's important to not skip any meals, skimp on portions in the Lean & Green Meal, or exercise too much while following the 5 & 1 Plan.

You can enjoy up to 45 minutes of vigorous exercise such as cardiovascular activity, resistance training, intense yoga, or Pilates each day while you're in the weight-loss phase. Medifast recommends this amount of exercise to create the right caloric deficit for weight loss without causing your body to conserve its energy stores.

When you follow the 5 & 1 Plan as directed and eat all five Medifast Meals, along with correct portions of your Lean & Green Meal, you're getting all the nutrition you need in terms of protein, carbohydrates, vitamins, minerals, and overall calories.

The benefits of physical activity

Physical activity supports a healthy lifestyle in myriad ways. It helps you maintain a healthy body weight, improves your overall health and fitness, and reduces your risk for many chronic diseases. Regular exercise improves your mood and outlook, strengthens your cardiovascular and pulmonary systems, and builds your muscular strength and endurance. Plus, it's fun! Physical activity is a great way to let go of stress and enjoy time with family, friends, or co-workers.

It's easy to start: Think in terms of incorporating exercise and physical activities into your daily life. Walking the dog, taking the stairs instead of the elevator, and parking the car farther away from your destination are just some examples of getting more physical motion into your life. And they all burn calories and help you maintain a healthy body weight. But don't stop there: Regular, structured exercise is important, too; you'll burn calories and improve your overall fitness level and health.

Cardiovascular, muscle strengthening and endurance, and flexibility activities are the three core components to a healthy exercise regimen.

Cardiovascular exercise

The cardiovascular (also known as "cardio" or aerobic) portion of your workout strengthens your heart and lungs. Regular cardio activity maximizes your heart's ability to pump your blood and deliver oxygen and nutrients through blood vessels. And when your lungs are performing optimally, you are trading off oxygen and carbon dioxide efficiently to make breathing during exercise easier. The two systems work together to deliver nutrient- and oxygen-rich blood to your working muscles during exercise sessions, and also throughout the day as you move your body. As you increase your fitness level, you'll notice that exercise and movement become easier. Cardio includes any activity that elevates your heart rate, including brisk walking, jogging, riding a bike, swimming, aerobic exercise classes, tennis, and basketball.

Strength training

Lean muscle mass is a metabolically active tissue: The more you have, the more calories you can burn, even at rest. Muscular strength training enables you to condition your muscles' exercise performance for maximal power. As you develop muscular strength, you'll benefit from increased endurance, which allows you to work your muscles for extended periods of time with less fatigue. Both strength and endurance are key ingredients for overall health, and greatly benefit your bone health, metabolism, and connective tissue strength—as well as cutting down your risk of injury.

Lifestyle exercise

A well-rounded and well-designed exercise program will also improve your flexibility—the ability of your body's joints to accommodate pain-free movement. Being flexible does not mean being able to twist like a pretzel; it is about optimal range of motion in all joints of the body. Static stretching involves a slow, gradual, and controlled elongation of the muscle through its full range of motion. A strong flexibility program in your workout yields a reduced risk of injury, improved posture, increased nutrient delivery to muscles, better balance within muscle groups, and improved performance.

The right amount of exercise for weight loss and weight maintenance

Several professional organizations have agreed on a set of guidelines for how much exercise is optimal for your overall fitness level and health. These guidelines, known as "FITT," also apply to weight loss and maintenance.

FITT is an acronym that stands for Frequency (how often you work out), Intensity (level of challenge), Time (duration of your workout), and Type of exercise. The FITT principle helps you track your exercise program and gives you a framework of clear goals with which to measure your progress. FITT can apply to all three components of your fitness program: cardiovascular, muscular strength, and flexibility. Let's look at each individually:

Table 1. FITT – Guidelines for optimal overall fitness

Program Component	F: Frequency	I: Intensity	T: Time	T: Type
Cardiovascular exercise	3 to 6 days per week	A certain heart rate range or rating of perceived exertion. *This is explained in more detail later in this chapter.*	20 to 60 minutes of aerobic activity daily. Exercise sessions can be broken down into 10-minute segments.	Any activity that involves large muscle groups.
Examples of cardiovascular exercise: Walking, biking, swimming, playing tennis, stair climbing, running, hiking, or playing basketball.				

Program Component	F: Frequency	I: Intensity	T: Time	T: Type
Muscular/ strength training	2 to 3 days per week	**For strength:** 1-3 sets of 8-12 repetitions at a weight that allows full range of motion to the point of temporary muscular fatigue. **For endurance:** Try pushing yourself to perform 1-3 sets of 10-15 repetitions.	Enough time to perform 1-3 sets of exercises for 8-10 major muscle groups (approximately 30 to 60 minutes).	· Free weights · Resistance tubing · Select equipment (Nautilus®, Cybex®, Life Fitness®, etc.) · Or your own body weight (e.g., pushups)
Examples of muscular/strength training: Chest presses using a barbell, shoulder presses using dumbells, leg presses using a leg press machine, pushups using your body weight, or bicep curls using resistance tubing.				
Flexibility	2 to 7 days per week	Stretch to the point of mild discomfort.	10-30 seconds for each static stretch	Static stretching involving all major muscle groups.
Examples of flexibility training: Stretch your chest, back (upper and lower), shoulders, legs (upper and lower), and arms.				

Nautilus® is a registered trademark of Nautilus, Inc. Cybex® is a registered trademark of Cybex International, Inc. Life Fitness® is a registered trademark of Brunswick Corporation.

The intensity of your exercise

Exercising at the right level of intensity is key to improving your overall fitness level and burning calories, while making the most efficient use of your time. You can measure the intensity of your cardiovascular exercise sessions two ways: Estimated target heart rate range or perceived exertion scale.

Estimated target heart rate range

When it comes to gauging the intensity of your cardiovascular exercise session, listen to your BPM—that's beats per minute. Your heart rate will tell you if you are working too hard, at an appropriate level, or not hard enough.

A particular range of BPM signals that your body is working at the right intensity level for sustained exercise and improved fitness. The goal while exercising is to stay within this heart rate range for a safe and effective session that improves your cardiovascular health.

Here's how to estimate your own target heart rate:

1. The first step is determining your age-based maximum heart rate, or MHR. Simply subtract your age from 220. (So, for example a 42-year-old woman would have a theoretical maximum heart rate of 178 BPM.)

2. Your target heart rate range for cardiovascular exercise is 55 percent to 90 percent of your MHR. (You get a range to allow for varying levels of intensity).

If you are just starting an exercise program or have a heart condition, your physician may recommend you begin exercising at 55 percent to 60 percent of your MHR. But if your heart is healthy and you are fairly active, exercising at 60 percent to 80 percent of your MHR may be a good place to begin.

It's easy to measure your heart rate. You can buy a heart rate monitor that you wear while exercising, or you can use the heart rate sensors on various pieces of exercise equipment. You can even measure your heart rate with your hand. Use your index and middle fingers, and place them gently on the pulse point, then count the number of beats that you feel in one minute—or, count the beats for 30 seconds and multiply that number by two.

Finding pulse points is easy. The two most accessible ones are the carotid artery (in your neck) or the radial artery (in your wrist). You'll find your carotid artery on the right side of your neck, just to the right of the center. You can locate it by moving your index and middle fingers from the inside to the outside of your right eyebrow and then drag your fingers across your face and to the middle of your neck until you can feel the pulse point.

Your radial artery pulse point is at the base of your thumb on the inside of the wrist. Place your hand palm side up, drag your index and middle fingers along your thumb toward your wrist, and you'll find the point where you feel your pulse.

Calculating estimated target heart rate ranges for exercise

Suzie is a 53-year-old woman who wants to calculate her exercise intensity for her cardiovascular workouts. First Suzie has to calculate her target heart rate range.

Step 1: Suzie estimates her MHR by subtracting her age from 220.

220 – 53 = 168 BPM.

Step 2: Suzie finds her exercise range (55 percent to 90 percent of her MHR).

168 x .55 (55 percent) = 92.4 or 93 BPM

168 x .90 (90 percent) = 151.2 or 152 BPM

Suzie's target heart rate range is 93 to 152 BPM, which means that when she's doing any cardiovascular exercise, she wants to ensure her exercising heart rate stays in that range to improve her fitness level. As Suzie gets more and more physically fit, she can stay at the higher end of this range for longer periods of time.

Remember—these are estimates. If you feel you are exercising too hard, you probably are. Make sure you're working out within a heart rate range that is challenging, but comfortable for you. As your fitness level improves, you can move your goal toward the higher end of your calculated target heart rate range.

Please note: If you are taking medications called beta blockers, using a target heart rate range is not recommended. That's because these medications are designed to slow your heart rate, so this method to measure intensity may not be accurate. Medifast suggests that clients on beta blockers use the Rate of perceived exertion method (below) instead.

Rate of perceived exertion scale

This scale was created in the 1950s by Dr. Grunnar Borg, and is sometimes referred to as the Borg Scale. It takes into consideration psychological, cardiovascular, musculoskeletal, and environmental factors and their effects on exercise intensity.

The original scale was based on a numerical rating that went from six to 20; however, it's since been revised to a numerical rating of zero to 10. You can use either scale.

Table 2. Rating of Perceived Exertion (RPE)

6 to 20 Borg Scale		0 to 10 Borg Scale	
6		0	nothing at all
7	very, very light	0.5	very, very weak
8		1	very weak
9	very light	2	weak
10		3	moderate
11	fairly light	4	somewhat strong
12		5	strong
13	somewhat hard	6	
14		7	very strong
15	hard	8	
16		9	
17	very hard	10	very, very strong
18			
19	very, very hard		
20			

To improve your fitness level, you want to work toward a range of 12 to 16 on the six to 20 Borg scale, or four to five on the zero to 10 version.

A good level of intensity is just as important for the muscular strength/endurance portion of your exercise program. To improve your fitness level when performing strength training exercises, you need to challenge yourself with enough weight or resistance to work your muscles to the point of temporary fatigue with each set. In other words, the last few repetitions of your strength exercises should be tough to finish.

Intensity is important in your flexibility program, too. You should stretch using a slow, smooth motion to a point in the stretch where you feel a slight discomfort. Hold the stretch at this point for 10 to 30 seconds, and you'll find that over time, as your flexibility improves, your stopping point will change.

Making progress

As you reach a healthy body weight and become more fit, your exercise sessions will become easier. When you have reached a point where the workout is easy or too easy, it's time to change it up a bit so you're still challenged. You can choose to increase the intensity, boost the duration, or try a new activity.

Try dialing up to a higher level of intensity or a higher speed on pieces of equipment such as a treadmill, elliptical machine, or stair climber. If you're taking group exercise classes, try a class at the next level up—for example, if you are currently taking classes at the beginner level, try an intermediate class.

Making even small adjustments in the intensity, duration, or type of exercise is a great way to advance your fitness level and overall health. Just be careful not to overdo it, and take it slow. (It is recommended to progress either exercise intensity or duration, but not both at the same time.) Exercising beyond your intensity or duration abilities, or trying new activities beyond your fitness level, can cause injury—and bring your entire fitness program to a temporary halt.

Where to exercise

Most overweight people aren't comfortable with the idea of going to a gym and being surrounded by a bunch of hard-bodied people. While there are some health clubs that cater to these super-fit types, plenty of fitness centers and health clubs are frequented by people of all shapes, sizes, and fitness levels.

If you're lucky enough to have a fitness center or health club in your area where you feel comfortable, go for it. You'll be able to work with state-of-the-art equipment and try out various types of activities such as racquetball, basketball, swimming, group exercise classes, and even complimentary programming such as yoga (which is great for both strength and flexibility).

Health clubs also tend to hire knowledgeable staff who can help you set up an exercise program that's a good fit for your age, health, and fitness level. When consulting with any health club staff or trainers, make sure they have a college degree in exercise science or a related field, or hold a current personal trainer certification from a recognized organization. Your best bet is a trainer who has completed a National Commission for Certifying Agencies-accredited certification.

If gyms and fitness centers aren't for you, you can still exercise in the comfort of your own home, your backyard, or a nearby park. As long as you feel safe and comfortable, it doesn't matter where you exercise—what matters is incorporating a regular exercise plan into your life and sticking to it.

Finding time to exercise

One of the biggest excuses for not exercising regularly is lack of time. And it's justified—most people's hectic schedules have them tied up with work, business, and family obligations, not to mention keeping up with the house work and yard work.

Carving out time for healthy fitness can be tough, but it's not impossible. Take a close look at your time and try these suggestions:

- Schedule exercise into your day like you would a business or doctor's appointment. You wouldn't cancel a meeting with others, so don't let anything cancel a meeting with yourself.
- Talk a walk during your break or lunch time. It's a great way to visit with friends or co-workers, and it's less expensive than going out to lunch. Most people find themselves more productive at work following an exercise break.
- Wake up a bit earlier and take a walk or pop in an exercise DVD. Start your day off with health while others are still sleeping.
- Trade off a babysitting hour with a neighbor. Your neighbor can babysit while you exercise, then you can return the favor.
- Look at your daily schedule and find ways to fit in shorter bouts of

exercise such as several 10-minute sessions throughout your day. You can still get results!

- Fit exercise into your play and social time. Get your kids involved with playing games of tag, leapfrog, jump rope, or hopscotch. Turn social visits into exercise visits. If you normally meet a girlfriend for coffee, try going for a walk. Instead of going to a movie, try bowling.

Special considerations

Check with your physician before starting any exercise program, especially if you have any medical history, including:

- Heart, lung, or kidney disease
- High blood pressure, high cholesterol, diabetes, arthritis, asthma, or osteoporosis
- Prescription medications
- Joint pain, injuries, or replacement surgery
- Any family history of heart disease before age 55.

Listen to your body when exercising. Some days you will feel better than others; you can adjust your exercise program accordingly. Although most people will have no problems with exercise, some issues require medical attention. If you experience any of the following, you should STOP your exercise sessions and consult your physician before resuming your exercise program:

- Nausea
- Dizziness or light-headedness
- Unusual or severe fatigue
- Severe leg pain or cramps
- Severe shortness of breath.

NOTE: If you experience any chest pain or pain in the arms, neck, jaw, or upper back, stop exercising immediately. If the pain lasts longer than two minutes after stopping the session, seek medical attention immediately. If the pain subsides, consult your physician before resuming your exercise program.

Yield to weather conditions

If you choose to exercise outdoors during hot and humid or cold weather conditions, you'll need to heed some precautions to stay safe:

On hot and humid days:

1. Exercise in the early morning or later in the evening when it is cooler.
2. Drink extra fluids.
3. Wear loose, lightweight, moisture-wicking clothing.
4. Stop immediately if you feel dizzy, lightheaded, or nauseated.
5. Adjust the intensity and duration of your exercise accordingly.

On cold days:

1. Wear layers of absorbent clothing. As you exercise and your body warms up, you can remove layers as needed to avoid overheating. Clothes that wick moisture away from the body will help keep your body surface dry and warm.
2. Be sure to cover your head and hands for protection from the elements and heat loss.
3. Stop immediately if you feel dizzy, lightheaded, or nauseated.
4. Adjust the intensity and duration of your exercise accordingly.

Exercise is beneficial on so many levels, and is a great way to feel stronger, more confident, and less stressed—plus, you'll burn plenty of calories! With all these great advantages, what are you waiting for? Make the commitment to yourself and your health, and get moving!

Shannon Wollam

lost 75 pounds with Medifast

"THANK YOU MEDIFAST! I am so grateful for the Medifast Program. This Program has allowed me to focus on why I eat instead of what I eat by taking the guesswork out of meal preparation.

"I have been heavy most of my life. I have yo-yoed back and forth so many times; tried sssssooo many diet plans, etc. but never did I change my eating habits or want to discover why I was eating.

"I am part of a cosmetic field and looking put together is very important. I certainly wasn't cute and put together. I was wearing a size 20 suit jacket and a size 22 skirt. I was having trouble with my breathing and the most embarrassing thing was when I noticed I was having trouble fitting in an airplane seat. I had enough!

"On the Medifast Program, you just eat when you're told to, eat what you're told to, and exercise and drink water and start to move your body. When you lose the weight, you gain confidence, and you gain another block you can walk, another lap you can swim.

"I am so enjoying being able to move again. I'm swimming, walking (2 miles a day), lifting weights, doing almost anything I can get my hands on. I love being in my body again! Medifast has changed my life. I will be forever grateful for that."

Results will vary.

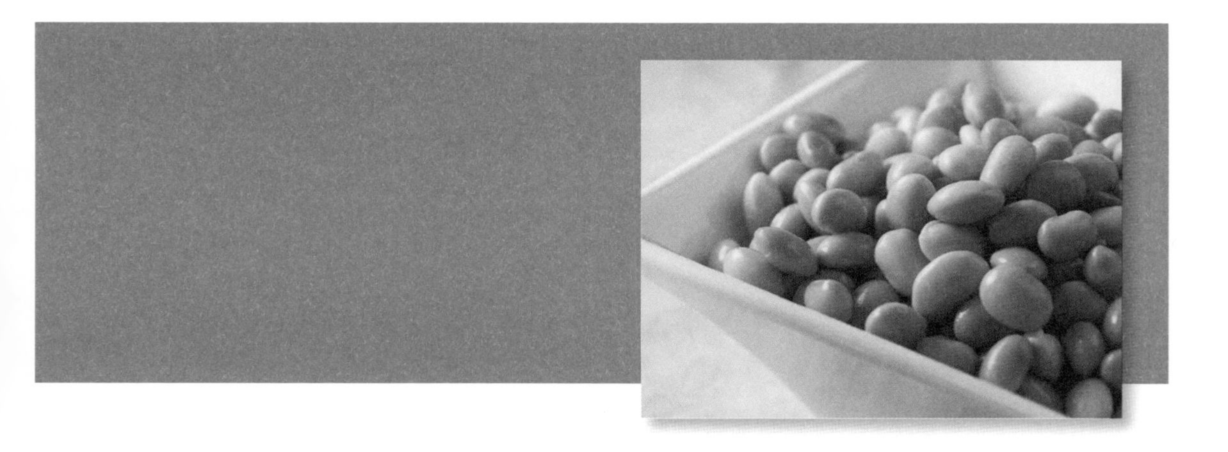

9 Soy and your health

Discovering the truth

The Medifast Program is based on a diet of foods that are high-protein, low-carbohydrate, and low-fat. One food satisfies all these conditions, and is the basis of most Medifast Meals: soy. Results of human and animal studies show that soy offers a number of additional health benefits, ranging from protection against cardiovascular disease and cancer to overall longer life.

Many weight-loss programs center on a diet rich in protein, and with good reason. Protein is the most satiating kind of food—that is, eating it makes you feel more full and satisfied than eating carbohydrates or fats. It takes longer for the body to break down protein and use it for fuel than it does to break down fats or carbohydrates. Eating foods rich in lean protein allows you to lose weight without losing lean muscle mass.

Yet all protein is not created equal. When you're trying to lose weight you may find that protein from some forms of meat may be higher in fat (including unhealthy saturated fat) than vegetable-based protein such as soy. Also, some people are conscious of the environmental impact of meat production, and others are concerned about the safety and ethics of eating meat.

Soy is a great source of protein, equal in quality to protein from meat, milk, and eggs. It is especially nutritious when processed correctly. Medifast Meals are made from very high-quality isolated soy protein, which is extracted from soybeans using a water-based technique that separates the beans protein from the carbohydrates and fat. The protein isolation process is important because it preserves the soybeans naturally occurring isoflavones—nutrients that are responsible for certain health benefits particular to soy. Lower-quality soy protein is extracted using alcohol, which removes a large amount of the isoflavones.

Health benefits

Soy in Japan

According to the Health and Welfare Statistics Association, the Japanese as a people live longer than anyone else in the world. Soy is a staple in the Japanese diet, and a study of 28,000 Japanese men and women over a seven-year period shows a relationship between eating soy and a lower chance of dying from any cause.[33]

Cardiovascular health

Soy lowers the risk for heart disease in several ways, particularly in lowering harmful cholesterol that can cause blockages in the blood vessels of the heart.

In 1999, the U.S. Food and Drug Administration (FDA) declared, based on 27 different studies, that eating foods high in soy protein is beneficial for the cardiovascular system. The isoflavones in soy protect the heart by helping to cleanse the bloodstream of LDL (bad) cholesterol and increasing the amount of HDL (good) cholesterol. Many Medifast Meals contain enough soy to earn the official "heart-healthy" label.

Soy also has anti-oxidant and anti-inflammatory properties that can support healthy aging and prevent wear-and-tear on the cells of the heart and blood vessels. Research has also shown that eating soy lowers levels of homocysteine, an amino acid that is associated with heart disease.

Metabolic syndrome

An increasing number of people from developed countries are being diagnosed with metabolic syndrome, and as a result are at risk for serious health problems such as type 2 diabetes and heart disease.

Metabolic syndrome is a cluster of health problems centering on how you metabolize food; that is, how you break down its components and use it for energy. The syndrome includes excess fat in the abdomen, fat in the bloodstream, high blood pressure, and a resistance to insulin, the hormone from the pancreas that helps break down sugars. The body also becomes prone to inflammation, which contributes to disease as we learned in chapter 5. Its exact cause isn't known, but diet is thought to play a key role in the development of metabolic syndrome.

Research on humans and animals shows that regularly eating soy protein can protect the body from developing metabolic syndrome. Soy foods can help to balance the metabolic system so your body can use insulin properly to regulate blood sugar.[34-36]

Prostate cancer

Obese men are more likely to die from cancer of the stomach or prostate than are non-obese men. And American men die of prostate cancer 18 times more often than Asian men. It's not merely a matter of genetics; even Asian men who come to the U.S. and adopt a typical American diet have a higher chance of dying of prostate cancer than those who stick with a traditional Asian, soy-intensive diet. In another study, mice that were fed a diet high in soy showed less prostate growth, which may mean less chance of cancer.

Breast cancer

Studies of breast cancer rates show a similar pattern. Asian women get breast cancer at a rate of 39 per 100,000, while 133 out of 100,000 Western women develop the disease.[37] Yet, when Asian women emigrate to the U.S., their chances of developing breast cancer increase substantially. This pattern seems to apply particularly to women who have not yet reached menopause.

The National Cancer Institute (NCI) recognizes that several studies show that eating soy may reduce the risk of getting breast cancer, and can improve chances of survival for those who do get the disease. However, some breast tumors (and the drugs used to treat them) react differently to the hormone-like isoflavones found in soy. NCI stresses that it does not recommend that breast cancer patients try to prevent a recurrence of the disease by eating soy protein. In the case of any disease, especially a serious one, it's essential to follow the advice of your physician.

Digestive system cancer

Five research studies show that eating soy regularly is associated with lower rates of cancer affecting the esophagus (the tube leading from the mouth to the stomach), the stomach, and the intestines.[38-41] Also, research shows that eating soy seems to lower the chance of becoming ill from Helicobacter pylori, a bacterium that is linked to stomach ulcers and stomach cancer.[42] Finally, numerous studies show a relationship between regular soy consumption and lower cell growth in the colon, including people with polyps of the colon, which can turn cancerous.

Menopausal symptoms

Two-thirds of women experience hot flashes and night sweats during menopause. Other women going through the "change of life" may have trouble concentrating or experience mood swings. The isoflavones in soy can make a difference in all of these symptoms, and eating soy regularly may help some women avoid having to go on prescription hormone replacement therapy. Most important, the high protein and low fat content of soy can help women avoid extra pounds—and associated health risks—during and after menopause.

Bone loss

Women start to lose bone mass rapidly after menopause due to the decline in estrogen. Brittle bones can set the stage for fractures and immobility, and a general decline in health and quality of life. Numerous experiments have shown that the isoflavones in soy can strengthen bones and slow bone loss. This effect may be seen more in women approaching menopause or in their early post-menopausal years, rather than women whose menopause is further advanced.

The safety of soy

It's important to get the straight facts about soy protein and how safe it is for your diet. Scientific studies reveal the following about soy and its relationship to certain health issues:

Thyroid medicine

People taking synthetic thyroid hormones may safely eat soy three hours before or after taking their medication. If you are on these meds and eating a lot of soy, be sure to tell your doctor, and work with him or her to closely monitor your thyroid levels. (Medifast Meals provide you with adequate amounts of iodine, a nutrient that's important to normal thyroid function.)

Fertility

Eating soy over the long term has no effect on child or adult growth, development, or sexual behavior. Soy may provide a slight decrease in testosterone levels, which may protect males from prostate cancer, and does not affect male fertility.

Kidney stones

Soy foods may contain an ingredient (oxalate) that may be of concern to people prone to getting calcium oxalate kidney stones. However, the superior processing of the soy protein that goes into Medifast products ensures that even when you are eating five soy-based Medifast Meals per day, you are only getting a fraction of the American Dietetic Association's recommended limit for people who tend to form calcium oxalate kidney stones.

For most people, the benefits of incorporating soy protein into a healthy diet far outweigh what little risk is involved. Remember, being overweight or obese is a potentially dangerous health condition that responds well to soy-based foods. Medifast is a pioneer in applying the benefits of high-quality soy protein that's rich in isoflavones and a great source of nutrition for lifelong weight control and general health.

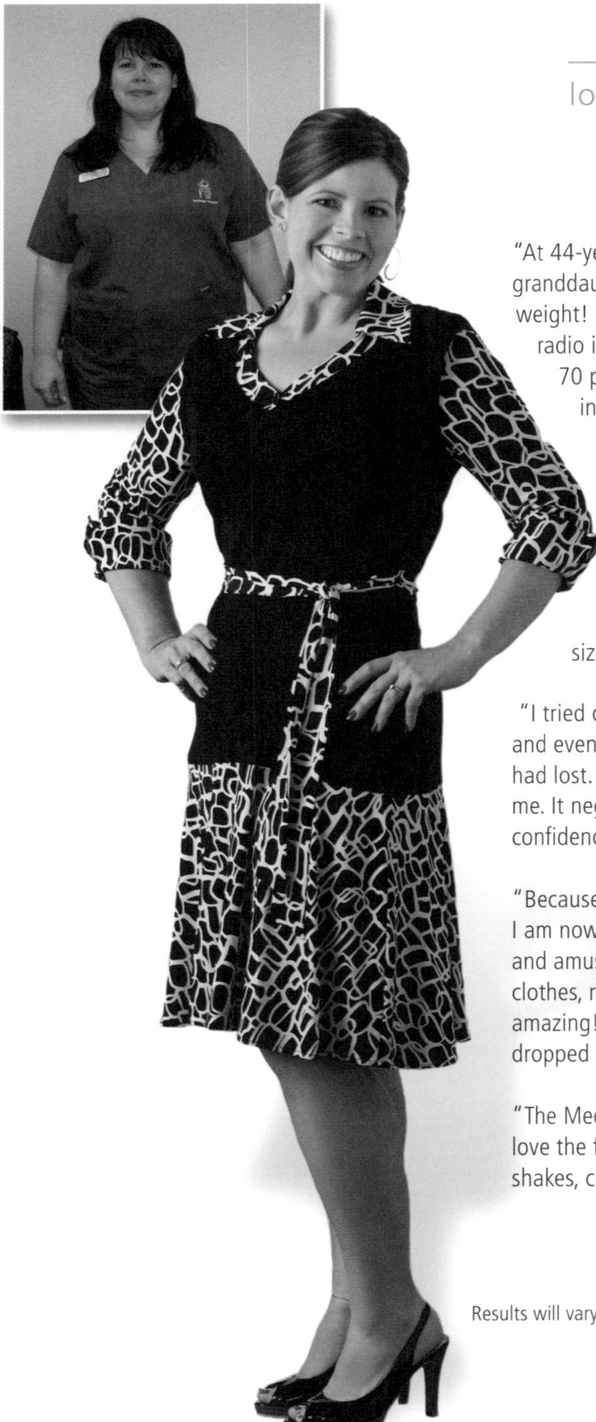

Tanya Sexton

lost 82 pounds with Medifast

"At 44-years-old with four children and a granddaughter on the way, I knew I needed to lose weight! My mother was listening to K-LUV morning radio in Dallas and heard that DJ Cathy Jones lost 70 pounds on Medifast and suggested I look in to it.

"I made an appointment and started with Medifast in February 2006 weighing 243 pounds, and in the first 2 weeks I lost 14 pounds! Here I am 64 weeks later and I have lost a total of 82 pounds, 12 inches off my waist, and I dropped 5 pant sizes.

"I tried other diets but didn't stick with them and eventually gained back double the amount I had lost. Being overweight took a lot away from me. It negatively affected my health and my self-confidence. It also affected my social and work life.

"Because of my success on the Medifast Program, I am now able to fit into chairs, airplane seats, and amusement park rides. I am able to wear cute clothes, run faster, and jump higher—it's absolutely amazing! I regulated my thyroid and my cholesterol dropped 29 points.

"The Medifast Program has been easy and fast. I love the food, especially the chocolate pudding, shakes, chicken noodle soup, and the bars."

Results will vary.

This success story lost weight using a Medifast Weight Control Centers Program.

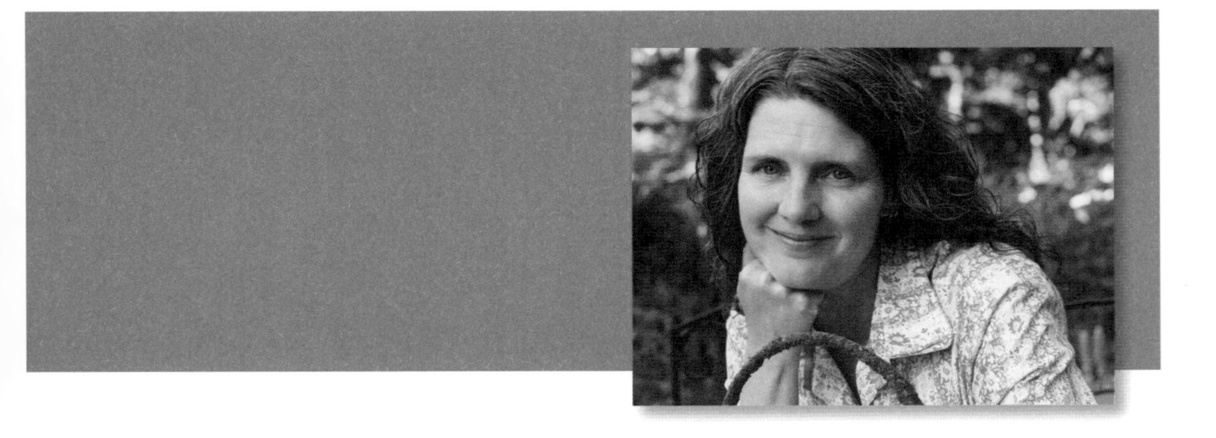

10 Medifast for Women's Health

When it comes to dieting and weight loss, women are the ones who traditionally seek out diets. There are many diets out there, and a large percentage of women have tried and failed many of them. Women generally know a lot about nutrition and dieting, yet struggle with losing the extra pounds and keeping them off.

This chapter was designed to help women succeed in losing weight on Medifast. It begins by having you take a closer look at what motivates you. It will help you to identify current or previous reasons for not losing weight, and offer some practical solutions.

This chapter will also address specific health conditions that affect women and reveal how Medifast's nutritionally enhanced foods can help. Because women's body weight and health issues often change as they move through the life cycle, this chapter will discuss how Medifast can meet both the dietary and health needs of pre- and post-menopausal women.

Motivational tactics

In general, there are some inherent differences between men and women in what motivates them when it comes to losing weight. Determining what motivates you will help you succeed in losing weight and keeping it off. While men are generally motivated by personal challenge, intensity, and results, women are generally motivated by the following.

Appearance

We live in a society that values thinness, so it is not surprising that improving appearance is the most common reason women cite for wanting to lose weight. The influence of thinness on self-image seems to (unfairly) affect women more than it does men. While the desire to improve appearance can be very motivating, it tends to have a short-term effect, especially if you are losing weight to meet the expectations of others, or to gain acceptance from someone else. To have more of a long-term impact on your motivational level, you should be losing weight for YOU. It is also a good idea to have motivators other than appearance, as well.

Health

The idea of reducing health risks is certainly very important. Depending on the person and circumstances, this may be more motivating for some and less motivating for others. For instance, having your doctor advise you to lose weight so you don't have to start diabetes medication is likely more motivating than being told you "should" lose weight to prevent future health problems, like diabetes.

Social support and personal relationships

Women value social support and friendships. If you are a woman motivated by personal relationships, then consider ways of getting the emotional support you need through friends, a church or faith group, a Medifast personal coach, or a personal trainer.

Medifast for women

Women of all ages frequently want to lose weight. Medifast has formulated three nutritionally enhanced lines of food (Medifast 55, Medifast 70, and Medifast Plus for Appetite Suppression) to meet the weight-loss and health needs of women of all ages. The following tables provide the nutritional facts about each.

Medifast 55

8g Soy protein Heart healthy	Calories	90	Kosher (dairy) Low-lactose Caffeine free* Contains whey
	Fat (g)	0-1	
	Saturated fat (g)	0	
	Protein (g)	11	
	Carbohydrate (g)	13-14	
	Fiber (g)	3-4	

Medifast 70

10g Soy protein Heart healthy	Calories	100	Kosher (dairy) Low-lactose Caffeine free* Contains whey
	Fat (g)	1	
	Saturated fat (g)	0	
	Protein (g)	14	
	Carbohydrate (g)	13-14	
	Fiber (g)	3-4	

Medifast Plus for Appetite Suppression

8.6-9g Soy protein Heart healthy	Calories	90	Kosher (dairy) Low-lactose Contains whey
	Fat (g)	1	
	Saturated fat (g)	0	
	Protein (g)	14	
	Carbohydrate (g)	11	
	Fiber (g)	4	
	Super Citrimax™ (mg)	300	

*Dutch Chocolate and Swiss Mocha flavors contain a small amount of caffeine.

Which nutritionally enhanced foods are right for me?

You may eat any combination of Medifast Meals on your program but Medifast has created these specific shakes to meet the needs of any individual. Let's take a look at some of their differences. Medifast 55 shakes were specifically formulated for women. The main difference between Medifast 55 and Medifast 70 is the protein content and total calories. Medifast 70 contains slightly more total protein and calories than Medifast 55, so women who are physically active might benefit from using Medifast 70. Medifast Plus for Appetite Suppression contains the same ingredients as Medifast 55, with the same protein content as Medifast 70, yet also contains the natural appetite suppressant, Super Citrimax™.

Super Citrimax™ is an all-natural plant extract derived from Garcinia cambogia, which is rich in hydroxycitric acid. Studies have demonstrated the effectiveness of Super Citrimax™ in weight management. Super Citrimax™ works by promoting the oxidative breakdown of fat, blocking the synthesis (or making of) fat, and by reducing brain levels of one of the most potent appetite-stimulating peptides called neuropeptide Y (NPY). Medifast Plus for Appetite Suppression is most appropriate for people who struggle with hunger and prefer the benefits of a natural appetite suppressant.

You may try any, or all, of the specialty products listed above. Mixing the meals may provide a greater variety and help you stay on your plan longer.

Medifast for menopausal (or peri-menopausal) women

Recognizing that female-related health issues begin to skyrocket after menopause, Medifast formulated Medifast Plus for Women's Health Shakes. These nutritionally enhanced meals were designed to aid in weight loss for women, ease the symptoms of menopause, and aid in fighting against female-related health conditions that tend to increase during this time (due to the loss of estrogen).

If you are an overweight woman just beginning to undergo the "change of life," or have been experiencing symptoms of menopause for quite some time, incorporating Medifast Plus for Women's Health Shakes into your program may be appealing to you as an alternative to, or in addition to, hormone replacement therapy (HRT).

If you are between the ages of 35 and 60, and are experiencing the symptoms of menopause/peri-menopause, Medifast Plus for Women's Health Shakes may be right for you. These shakes have been expressly formulated to meet the needs of menopausal women who want to lose weight. The following table summarizes some of the special ingredients Medifast uses to enhance the health of women undergoing the change. The table below show a more in-depth summary of each.

Medifast Plus for Women's Health Shakes

10g Soy protein Heart healthy	Calories Fat (g) Saturated fat (g) Protein (g) Carbohydrate (g) Fiber (g)	110 1 0 14 15 4	**Antioxidants:** Coenzyme Q10, pycnogenol **Botanicals:** Black cohosh, chaste tree berry, echinacea purpurea **Branched chain amino acids:** 1-leucine, 1-isoleucine, 1-valine Alpha lipoic acid, calcium

Medifast Plus for Women's Health Shakes provide as much protein as Medifast 70, contains the Super Citrimax™ appetite suppressant, plus have a host of health-enhancing ingredients to lessen the symptoms of menopause and reduce female-related health risks.

Health problems that affect women

Menopause/peri-menopause

Let's take a closer look at specific health concerns that affect women undergoing the change. Menopause is a normal biological event that occurs when a woman's ovaries stop producing female hormones and menstrual cycles come to an end. Most of the signs and symptoms of menopause result from a decrease in the amount of estrogen circulating in the bloodstream. Approximately two-thirds of women who reach menopause develop some degree of menopausal symptoms. Although the majority of women have some of these symptoms, menopause is not a disease, and for some may actually be a positive emotional and physical transition to the next stage of life.

The average age of menopause is 51. That means for today's typical western woman, she can expect to live at least one-third of her life in the post-menopausal phase. Additionally, many women have symptoms of peri-menopause for up to 10 years before having their final menstrual cycle. Have you been experiencing any of the signs and symptoms of menopause listed below?

Signs and symptoms of menopause/peri-menopause

- Hot flashes
- Numbness/tingling
- Heart palpitations
- Cold hands and feet
- Headaches
- Vertigo/dizziness
- Weight gain
- Painful intercourse
- Irritability
- Insomnia
- Anxiety
- Night sweats
- Nervousness
- Forgetfulness
- Depression
- Inability to concentrate
- Fatigue
- Vaginal dryness and decreased elasticity
- Increased fat deposits in lower abdomen, hips, and breasts

Below are the ingredients found in the Medifast Plus for Women's Health Shakes that may help alleviate the symptoms of menopause/peri-menopause.

Soy protein

Like other complete proteins, soy protein helps you gain metabolically active lean muscle mass, which burns more calories than tissue. Soy, however, may be superior to other proteins because it contains added health benefits. That is why almost all Medifast Meals are soy-protein based. Soy also contains estrogen-like compounds, termed isoflavones, which benefit menopausal women by providing small amounts of the estrogen that their bodies are no longer produce. Soy's isoflavones have antioxidant activity that can reduce the symptoms of menopause, and provide protection against heart disease, breast cancer, and osteoporosis.

One of the most commonly reported side effects of women undergoing the change is hot flashes. Hot flashes and night sweats are due to a loss of temperature control, one of the by-products of a slowed production of estrogen. Because of their estrogen-like effects, soy isoflavones may be an alternative way to control these symptoms. In Japan, where soy foods are commonly consumed daily, women are only one-third as likely to report peri-menopausal symptoms compared to women in the United States or Canada. In fact, there is no word in the Japanese language for "hot flashes."

Chaste Tree Berry (Vitex agnus castus)

Chaste Tree Berry is the fruit of a small Eurasian tree that has been used since ancient Greek times as a treatment for menstrual and peri-menopausal problems. It contains medicinally active components including flavonoids and iridoid glycodides (agnuside and aucubin). These active components act upon the pituitary gland in the brain, specifically on its production of luteinizing hormone, which influences progesterone levels during the luteal (or late) phase of the menstrual cycle.

Chaste tree berries may also affect the balance of female hormones (estrogen and progesterone) in the body indirectly by mimicking the brain neurotransmitter dopamine. By mimicking dopamine, chaste tree berries may also help to keep secretion of prolactin in check. Mildly elevated levels of prolactin are associated with breast pain and symptoms of premenstrual syndrome (PMS), such as abdominal bloating, cramping, irritability, and mood swings.

Black Cohosh (Cimicifuga racemosa)

Evidence to date suggests that black cohosh is a safe and effective way to reduce peri-menopausal symptoms, especially hot flashes. Clinical studies have shown that black cohosh also relieves a variety of other peri-menopausal complaints, from mood swings and depression to vaginal atrophy (inflammation and thinning of the vaginal lining and decreased lubrication).

Echinacea Purpura

Echinacea is the name of a genus of plants native to Midwestern North America, commonly known as the purple coneflower. Echinacea is commonly taken to alleviate symptoms of the common cold because it has been shown to reduce the severity and duration of upper respiratory tract symptoms. Because of its ability to boost the immune system, Echinacea may also be a useful agent in fighting off recurrent vaginal and bladder infections that occur during menopause.

Vitamin E succinate

Vitamin E is a fat-soluble vitamin with antioxidant activity that may reduce the frequency and severity of hot flashes. Also known for its moisturizing properties, vitamin E may help with vaginal dryness as well.

The benefits of Medifast Plus for Women's Health don't stop here. These meals may help decrease the incidence of health issues that affect menopausal women such as:

- Cardiovascular/Coronary artery disease
- Breast cancer
- Osteoporosis

Let's examine each of these health concerns more closely.

Coronary artery disease

Long thought of as a disease primarily affecting men, we now know that cardiovascular disease—including heart disease, hypertension, and stroke—also affects many women. The difference is that women generally develop heart disease about 10 to 15 years later than men, largely because, until menopause, they still have the cardio-protective effect of female hormones, like estrogen.

Cardiovascular disease is the leading cause of death among women in the United States and kills six times more women than breast cancer.[43] According to the Agency for Healthcare Research and Quality (AHRQ), one out of every two women will die of heart disease or stroke, and one out of 25 women will die of breast cancer.

The following are the ingredients found in the Medifast Plus for Women's Health Shakes that may help protect against coronary heart disease.

Soy protein

Since estrogen helps protect against heart disease, women are at greater risk for heart problems after menopause (when estrogen levels decline). The isoflavones found in soy provide small amounts of estrogen that may protect against heart disease. Dozens of controlled clinical studies have shown that foods rich in soy protein are good for heart health. Soy protein has been shown to lower levels of total cholesterol, low-density lipoprotein LDL (bad cholesterol), and triglycerides without affecting the amount of high-density lipoprotein HDL (good cholesterol). Soy is so effective at doing this, it has earned the health claim: "heart-healthy." According to the U.S. Food and Drug Administration (FDA), diets containing 25g/day of soy may reduce total cholesterol levels, in particular, LDL levels.

Vitamin E

Antioxidants like vitamin E may protect your cells against free radicals, which are potentially damaging by-products of energy metabolism. Free radicals may lead to cardiovascular disease and cancer. Free radicals cause the oxidation of LDL cholesterol which is not good. Vitamin E may help prevent or delay cardiovascular disease/coronary heart disease by decreasing the oxidative effect of free radicals on LDL cholesterol. Vitamin E also may help prevent blood clots, which can lead to heart attacks. A study of approximately 90,000 nurses suggested that the incidence of heart disease was 30 to 40 percent lower among those with the highest intakes of vitamin E from diet and supplements.[44]

For more information about the cardio-protective effects of branched-chain amino acids, alpha lipoic acid, pycnogenol, and coenzyme Q10, please refer to Chapter 13.

Breast cancer

While heart disease is the biggest killer of American women, breast cancer is still a major cause for concern, especially in women who are overweight or obese. According to the American Obesity Association, there are significant weight-related risk factors for developing breast cancer:

- Post-menopausal women who are obese have a higher risk of developing breast cancer. In particular, gaining weight after menopause may increase breast cancer risk.

- Women who gain 45 pounds or more after age 18 are twice as likely to develop breast cancer after menopause than those whose weight remains stable.

Below are the ingredients found in Medifast Plus for Women's Health Shakes that may help protect against breast cancer.

Soy protein

Many of the compounds in soy have anti-cancer properties, but two types of isoflavones are particularly noteworthy, genistein and daidzein. Because isoflavones are weak estrogens, they appear to act as anti-estrogens by competing with the more potent, naturally occurring bodily estrogens for binding sites on estrogen receptors. This may explain why populations that consume high amounts of soy (e.g., Southeast Asia) have lower risks of estrogen-dependent breast cancer. Two human trials show that soy may decrease breast density and breast inflammation, two known risk factors for breast cancer.

Osteoporosis

Osteoporosis is a disease in which bones become thin, brittle and break easily. Many postmenopausal women are at increased risk of developing osteoporosis, especially if they are not taking hormone replacement therapy. The United States has one of the highest rates of osteoporosis in the world, affecting up to 25 percent of women. Like many women, you're probably concerned about your risk of osteoporosis. You may already be increasing your intake of dietary calcium, taking a calcium supplement, and/or using a prescription medication to prevent bone loss and decrease your risk of fracture. Research suggests another option for reducing bone loss is isoflavone-rich soy protein.

Below are the ingredients found in Medifast Plus for Women's Health Shakes that may help reduce the risk of osteoporosis.

Soy protein

The lumbar spine (lower back) is one of the places most susceptible to osteoporosis, and is also one of the most common sites for osteoporosis-related fractures in women at mid-life. Research has shown that after only six months of consuming 40g of soy protein high in isoflavones, bone loss in the low back was less in these women compared to women consuming 40g of whey-based protein. These results appear to be long lasting. A two-year study of postmenopausal women showed that isoflavone-rich soymilk prevented bone loss in the lumbar spine. Below are some reasons soy protein may protect bones.

- Some studies have shown that diets excessively high in animal protein cause more calcium to be leached from the bones and excreted in the urine and feces. In general, protein from soybeans does not have this effect on bone calcium. The extent to which protein actually affects bone heath is not fully known, but eating soy foods instead of animal protein may benefit the bones.
- Isoflavones in soy foods may actually inhibit the breakdown of bones. The isoflavone daidzein is very similar to the drug ipriflavone (used throughout Europe and Asia to treat osteoporosis). In fact, one of the byproducts of ipriflavone, when metabolized, is daidzein itself. Recent studies have also shown genistein may inhibit bone breakdown, and may have similar effects to estrogens in terms of maintaining bone tissue.
- Many soy foods are high in calcium (naturally or through fortification). In addition, soy also contains magnesium and boron, which are important co-factors of calcium for bone health.

Calcium/Vitamin D

Medifast Plus for Women's Health is fortified with three kinds of calcium; calcium citrate, calcium carbonate, and calcium phosphate. Calcium works with vitamin D to keep bones strong. Vitamin D is a fat-soluble vitamin that increases the absorption of calcium and phosphorus, which helps deposit these minerals in bones and teeth to keep them strong. Women who are deficient in calcium and vitamin D are at greater risk of osteoporosis and osteomalacia (softening of the bones).

If you are a woman, hopefully this chapter has provided you with the information and tools necessary to achieve your health and weight-loss goals with Medifast.

Denise Brown

lost 65 pounds with Medifast

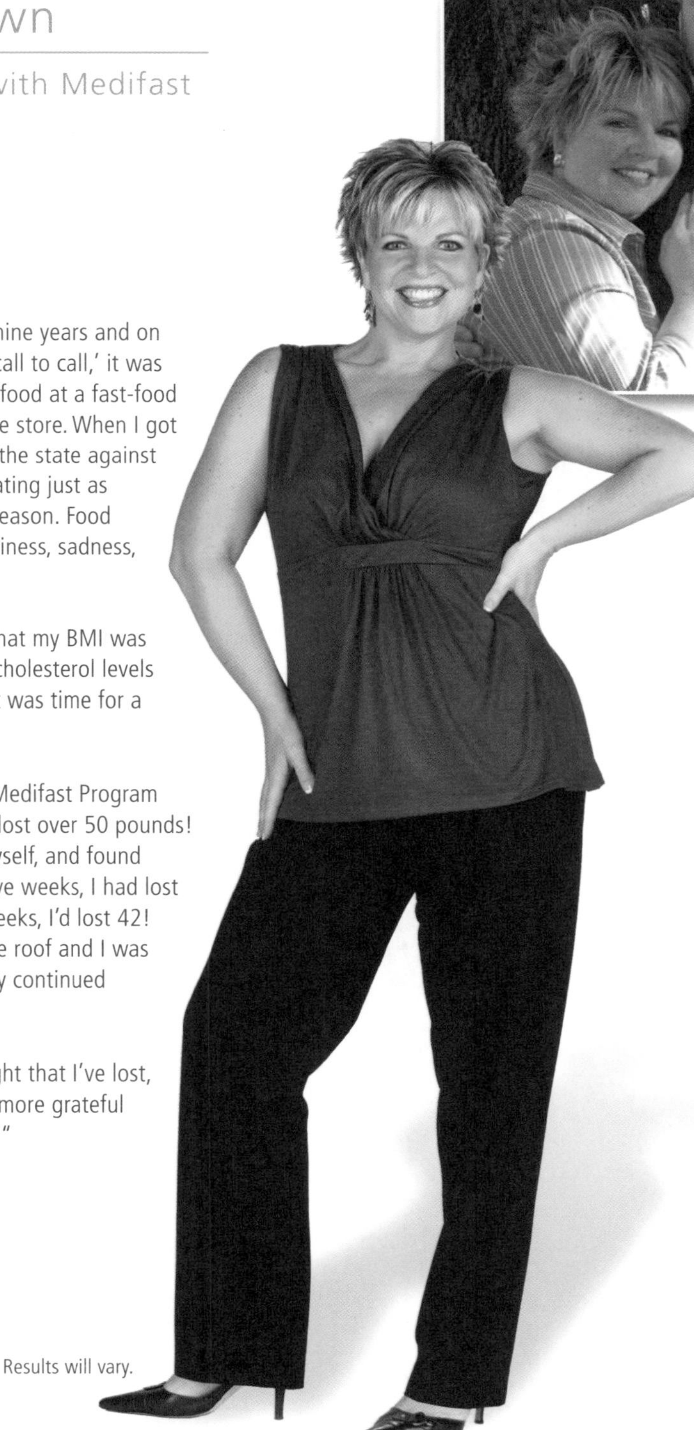

"I was a police officer for nine years and on those busy nights, racing 'call to call,' it was so much easier to stop for food at a fast-food restaurant or a convenience store. When I got my dream job working for the state against domestic violence, I was eating just as poorly, but for a different reason. Food was my comfort from loneliness, sadness, and boredom.

"My doctor informed me that my BMI was considered obese and my cholesterol levels were dangerously high—it was time for a change.

"That's when I found the Medifast Program through a friend who had lost over 50 pounds! I started the 5 & 1 Plan myself, and found great success! After just five weeks, I had lost 25 pounds and after 12 weeks, I'd lost 42! My energy was through the roof and I was constantly motivated by my continued results.

"I am grateful for the weight that I've lost, and kept off, but I'm even more grateful for having my health back."

Results will vary.

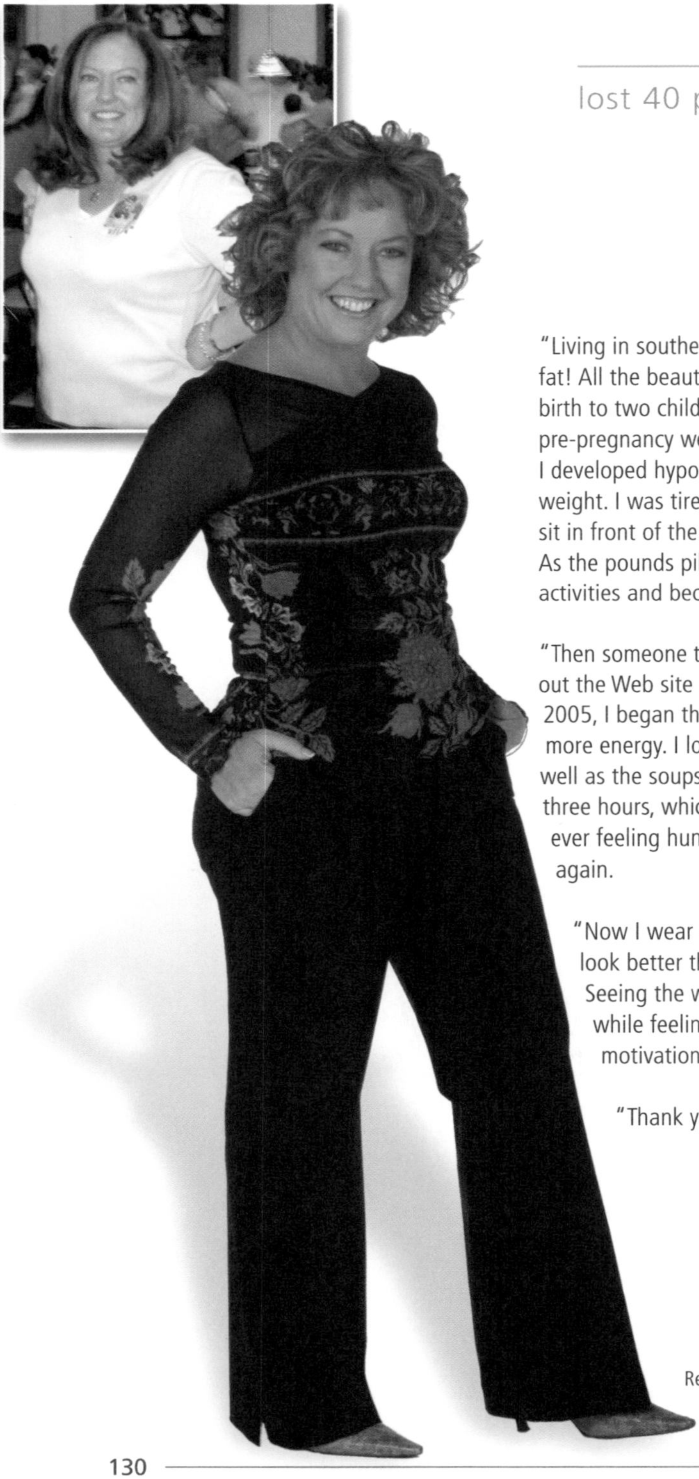

Kelly Ellis

lost 40 pounds with Medifast

"Living in southern Florida is not easy when you're fat! All the beautiful people are here! After giving birth to two children I was able to get back to my pre-pregnancy weight with diet and exercise. Then I developed hypothyroidism and began gaining weight. I was tired and not happy. All I could do was sit in front of the TV after a long day and munch. As the pounds piled on I had less interest in outside activities and became more run down.

"Then someone told me about Medifast. I checked out the Web site and loved what I saw. In October 2005, I began the Program and immediately I felt more energy. I love the oatmeal and the bars, as well as the soups and shakes. I was eating every three hours, which was great and kept me from ever feeling hungry. By December I was loving life again.

"Now I wear a size 6-8! I feel better and look better than I have in a very long time! Seeing the weight start to come off quickly, while feeling full and energetic, gave me the motivation I needed to change my life.

"Thank you Medifast!!"

Results will vary.

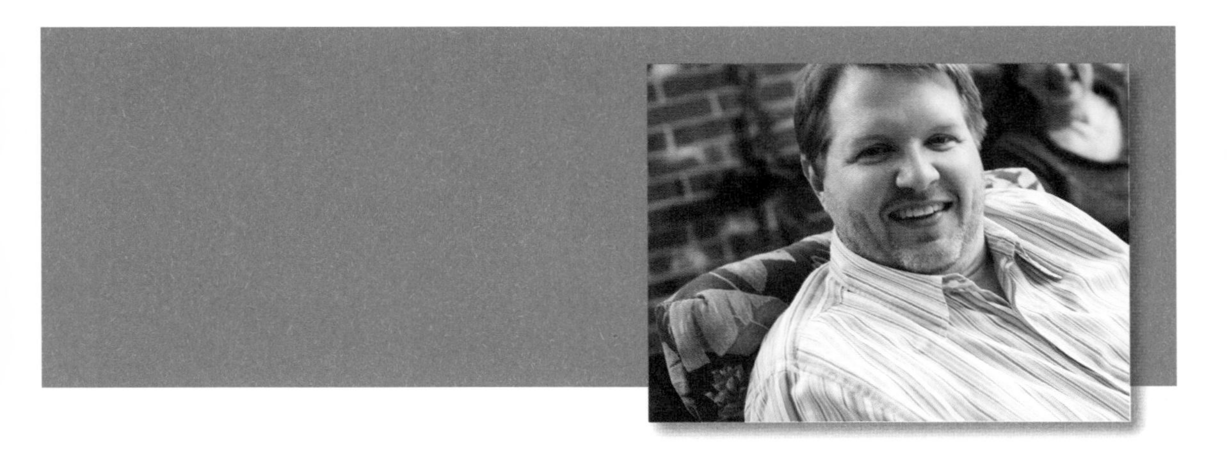

11 Medifast for Men's Health

When it comes to dieting and weight loss, men are often ignored. While it is women who traditionally seek out diets, the reality is that women are not the only ones who want (or need) to lose weight. Many men also wish they had trimmer waistlines, or are worried that their extra weight (particularly around the midsection) has associated health risks, like heart disease.

This chapter will help you succeed in your weight loss efforts on Medifast by having you take a closer look at what motivates you. It will also have you identify reasons you have had in the past, or currently have, for not losing weight, and offer some practical solutions.

This chapter will also look at specific health conditions that affect men as they go through the life cycle, and how specific ingredients in Medifast's nutritionally enhanced foods may improve health risks.

Motivational tactics

Let's begin with factors that motivate men. Men are unique, and as such, their motivation for wanting to lose weight generally differs from women. Men, as a whole, are notoriously bad at confronting their health issues proactively, so only when matters of serious concern like a heart attack, weakening erections, balding, or sport-related injuries occur, do men act. Paradoxically, the desire to improve their health or fitness level is often the number one reason given by men for wanting to lose weight.

Determining what motivates you as an individual will help you be successful in losing weight and keeping it off. Men tend to respond to different motivators than women when it comes to diet and exercise. While women tend to be more motivated by support (especially from family), men tend to be motivated more by the following:

Challenge

If you are a man that is motivated by challenge, then consider making a competition out of losing weight, perhaps with a spouse, friend, or co-worker. Start a competition where the guy who loses the most weight by a certain date wins. Make a bet. Wager something interesting (or humiliating) so that you will both be motivated to win, or at least not lose.

Results

If you are a man driven by results, then track ones that are important to you (e.g., weight, blood pressure, blood sugar) and monitor them on a regular basis. Be sure to write down or graph your progress. This can be highly motivating.

Support from friends

Men tend to respond better to support from friends rather than support from family. Men don't like to be nagged. If you are a man that responds to support from friends, get a weight-loss buddy to do it with you. Pick a friend who will push you in your weight-loss efforts.

Knowing what motivates you will help set the stage for your plan of action when it comes to losing weight with Medifast.

Medifast for men

Now that you have identified factors that motivate you (and identified what type of man you are when it comes to dieting and weight loss), let's look at how men can use Medifast's nutritionally enhanced foods to achieve their weight-loss goals. Medifast has created two lines to meet the weight-loss and health needs for men of all ages. The following tables provide the nutritional facts about each.

Medifast 70

10g Soy protein Heart healthy	Calories	100	Kosher (dairy) Low-lactose Caffeine free* Contains whey
	Fat (g)	1	
	Saturated fat (g)	0	
	Protein (g)	14	
	Carbohydrate (g)	13-14	
	Fiber (g)	3-4	

Medifast Plus for Men's Health

10g Soy protein Heart healthy	Calories	110	Kosher (dairy) Low-lactose Contains whey
	Fat (g)	1	
	Saturated fat (g)	0	
	Protein (g)	14	
	Carbohydrate (g)	15	
	Fiber (g)	4	
	Super Citrimax™ (mg)	300	

*Dutch Chocolate and Swiss Mocha flavors contain a small amount of caffeine.

Which nutritionally enhanced foods are right for me?

You may use any combination of Medifast Meals on your program. Because men (active men in particular) generally have slightly higher protein requirements than women do, Medifast has formulated these shakes to aid in your weight-loss efforts.

Health problems that affect men

Improving health is generally one of the major motivating factors behind weight loss for men. Losing just five to 15 percent of your body weight may improve your health and quality of life, get you off medications, and reduce your risk of future diseases. If you are a man who weighs 200 pounds, that means losing only 10 to 30 pounds may significantly reduce your risk of developing obesity-related diseases, or improve the status of already existing ones. In addition, the use of soy protein and other healthful ingredients found in Medifast's nutritionally enhanced foods may have added benefits for health conditions specific to men. These meals may help decrease the incidence of health conditions that affect men, such as:

- Cardiovascular/coronary artery disease
- Prostate cancer
- Erectile dysfunction
- Male-pattern baldness

This chapter will provide a general overview about health conditions that affect men, and how Medifast can help. The health-promoting components of Medifast's nutritionally enhanced foods are thoroughly described in Chapter 13, please refer to that chapter for more details.

Cardiovascular/coronary artery disease

According to the American Heart Association, men are at greater risk of having a heart attack than women, and they tend to have them earlier in life. Women are guarded against heart disease until menopause because of the protective effects of estrogen. Even after menopause, however, when women's death rate from heart disease increases, it is still not as great as men's. Below is the main ingredient found in Medifast Plus for Men's Health Shakes that may help protect against cardiovascular disease.

Soy protein

Soy protein is a complete protein that helps build metabolically active lean muscle mass, but also contains isoflavones that help even the playing field between men and women when it comes to heart disease. For men who have (or are at risk of developing) coronary artery disease, Medifast Plus for Coronary Health Shakes may be an option. Please see Chapter 13 for more information.

Soy contains two isoflavones, genistein and diadzein. These antioxidants protect against heart disease by slowing the growth of cells that form plaque in the coronary and other arteries. Since men are not blessed with estrogen's heart disease "protective" properties (by genetics), incorporating soy protein may help reduce their risk. Soy studies in men show that:

- Just 25 g/day of soy significantly reduces LDL (bad) cholesterol without affecting HDL (good) cholesterol.
- Low-fat diets high in soy protein (25 g/day) induce greater reductions in

total cholesterol, systolic blood pressure, and calculated cardiovascular disease risk compared to men on low-fat, but dairy (animal) protein diets.

Prostate Cancer

Men who are overweight have an increased risk of cancer. While lung cancer is the biggest killer among all men, overweight men who fall into the heaviest weight category are also more likely to die from stomach or prostate cancer, according to the American Cancer Society. The good news is that researchers have found that individuals with higher soy intakes have a lower risk of lung, stomach, and prostate cancer. Since prostate cancer is a major concern among many men, we will focus on that more in this section. Be aware that soy products may reduce the risk of other cancers as well.

Prostate cancer is the most common non-skin cancer among men in the United States, according to the American Cancer Society. Prostate cancer is the second biggest cancer killer of older American men, following lung cancer. One in six men will develop prostate cancer at some point in their lives.

American men are almost five times as likely to die of prostate cancer than Japanese men. Japanese men have some of the highest consumption rates of soy products worldwide, and have some of the lowest rates of prostate cancer. It is not that Japanese men never get prostate cancer, just that the high consumption of soy-based products (like tofu and soymilk) seems to delay the onset of cancer and slows the growth of their tumors. That is why the death rate for Japanese men from this disease is much lower than that of American men. The exception to this rule occurs when Japanese men migrate to the United States, and switch from a Japanese diet to a typical American diet. These Japanese men end up with similar prostate cancer death rates relative to their American counterparts.

Determining your risk

The following are risk factors for getting prostate cancer.

Age

The disease is rare in men younger than 45, but the chance of getting it goes up sharply as a man ages.

Family history

A man's risk of prostate cancer is higher if his father or brother has had the disease. A man with one close relative with the disease has double the risk. With two close relatives, his risk is five-fold. With three, the chance is 97 percent.

Race

Prostate cancer is more common in African-American men, and less common in Asian men.

Body weight

Men with a body mass index over 32.5 (obese range) have about a one-third greater risk of dying from prostate cancer than men who are not obese.

Benign Prostatic Hypertrophy (BPH)

Not to be confused with prostate cancer, BPH is a benign (non-tumor forming) enlargement of the prostate gland, likely due to testosterone in the gland. Most men over the age of 50 develop BPH. It may not cause any symptoms at all, or it may cause a number of urinary problems like increased frequency, hesitancy to urinate, and nighttime awakening to empty the bladder. Asian populations, who consume large amounts of soy, have been shown to also have a low incidence of BPH.

Male-pattern baldness

Twenty million men in the U.S. have male-pattern baldness. One in four men begin to go bald by age 30. Thirty percent of men are bald by age 55. And two out of three men are bald by age 60. In male-pattern baldness, when a hair falls out, a new one does not grow to replace it. This usually happens above the forehead, giving the familiar receding-hairline appearance. It also happens at the crown of the head. Over time, the bald spots increase in size until only the sides of the head are left with hair. If you want to know if you are likely to go bald, take a look at your mother's father to get your best guess. If he was bald, you are likely to be as well.

Why should I care about male-pattern baldness?

The main reason to care about male-pattern baldness is not a vanity reason. There is good evidence to suggest that baldness may be an indicator of both heart and prostate disease.

While baldness does not directly cause heart disease, the degree of baldness and the age at which baldness begins are strongly associated with the risk of heart disease. The common link between these two seemingly unrelated conditions is the male hormone testosterone. Men who lose their hair sooner, or to a greater extent, often have higher testosterone levels. These men also display higher conversion rates of testosterone to another male hormone, dihydrotesterone (DHT), which, among other actions, interferes with the growth of hair follicles. These two male hormones have been linked to heart disease risk factors like high blood pressure, elevated cholesterol, and hardening of the arteries. In fact, testosterone is one of the main reasons men have a higher risk of heart disease than women.

According to the Physicians Health Study, men with extensive baldness (that includes the crown of the head) and high cholesterol had a nearly 3-fold higher risk of heart disease than men with high cholesterol, but no hair loss. Men with extensive baldness and high blood pressure had an 80 percent increase in the risk of heart disease.[45]

Determining your risk

Brigham and Women's Hospital (a teaching affiliate of Harvard Medical School) studied the heart disease risk in men who are beginning to lose hair on the front of their heads. When compared to men with no hair loss at all, the risk of heart disease (nonfatal heart attacks, angina or chest pains, and procedures necessary to open blocked coronary arteries) increased by nine percent. When a bald spot appears on the crown, relative risk jumps 23 percent. When all hair is gone from the top of the head, the risk rises by a worrisome 36 percent. DHT also stimulates the growth of prostate cells, leading to BPH in many older men and may lead to prostate cancer. According to Australian researchers, men with bald spots at the top of their heads were one-and-a-half times more likely to have moderate to high-grade prostate cancer before age 70, than those without such bald spots.

Below are the ingredients found in Medifast Plus for Men's Health Shakes that may help protect against prostate disease and male pattern baldness.

Soy protein

Medifast foods are made mostly from soy protein, which has been shown to have a direct beneficial effect on the prostate gland. The isoflavones in soy have been shown to greatly reduce the risk of both BPH and prostate cancer. Soy has also been shown to help with male-pattern baldness. One of the isoflavones (genistein) has been shown to reduce the growth of prostate tissue.

Another soy isoflavone (daidzein) has been shown to stop the progression of prostate cancer and male pattern baldness by blocking the hormone DHT, which is known to stimulate prostate tissue growth. So, in addition to the weight-loss benefits, the use of soy protein (plus other prostate-friendly antioxidants in Medifast foods) may help reduce the risk of prostate cancer.

- Harvard University Medical School found that soy can drastically reduce tumor growth and its spread to other organs. Substances found in soybeans appear to block the development of blood vessels that are needed by tumors. Cutting off their blood and nutrient supply causes the tumors to starve to death.

In addition to soy, Medifast uses other prostate-friendly ingredients in its nutritionally enhanced meals, such as lycopene, selenium, zinc, and vitamins E and C. All but zinc are antioxidants that may help to reduce rates of prostate cancer by preventing the damage caused by free radicals. Zinc accumulates in the prostate gland, and may also have some protective properties against BPH and prostate cancer.

- Studies have shown that higher levels of selenium, vitamin E, and lycopene (found in tomato products), can help reduce the risk and progression of prostate cancer. Since most men fall short of getting the five or more servings of fruits and vegetables a day needed to get the protective effect of these antioxidants, Medifast proves to be a convenient solution.

Erectile dysfunction

If you're the type of guy who has a hard time getting motivated to lose weight, then consider that being overweight may be a cause of impotence. Let the prospect of a better sex life be a motivator for you to shed the extra pounds.

Thirty million men in the United States suffer from varying degrees of erectile dysfunction (ED). One study found that men who are overweight or obese (with a BMI of at least 28.7 kg/m2) have a 30 percent greater chance of ED than do lean men with a normal BMI (less than 25 kg/m2). Similarly, men with a 32-inch waistline were 50 percent less likely to have ED than men with a 42-inch waistline. Here are some ways that being overweight may be affecting your sex life:

- Mental and emotional issues that obesity can cause for intimacy
- Hormone imbalances

    Obesity is associated with lower testosterone levels and a higher conversion of male hormones to estrogen.

- Vascular disease

  The high rate of ED in men with cardiovascular disease suggests that vascular abnormalities of the arteries that supply blood to the penis play an important role in the development of ED. Men with CVD risk factors like diabetes, high cholesterol, and high blood pressure may have ED because of narrowing or blocking of the penile arteries.

Losing a little weight can do wonders for your sex life, according to a study at Duke University. Men and women who lost just 10 percent of their total body weight reported significant improvements in their sexual quality of life. One-third of obese, middle-aged (35 to 55 years) men with ED had significant improvements after two years of engaging in healthy behaviors, like regular exercise and weight loss.

At the very least, shedding a few pounds may improve intimacy by making people feel better about their bodies. Improving feelings of sexual attractiveness applies to men, too—not just women.

Just in case you were wondering if the plant estrogens in soy would interfere with your erectile function, the answer is no. Many studies have looked into the hormonal effects of soy intake on men, and none of them show any bad effects on sexual function. Perhaps more convincing are the thousands of male infants fed soy baby formula, who (as adults) have normal sexual function, testosterone levels, and semen quality.

In summary, Medifast is an excellent choice for men seeking to lower their health risks through weight loss, because it is specially formulated to address some of the most important health concerns affecting men. It is also easy to use and satisfying.

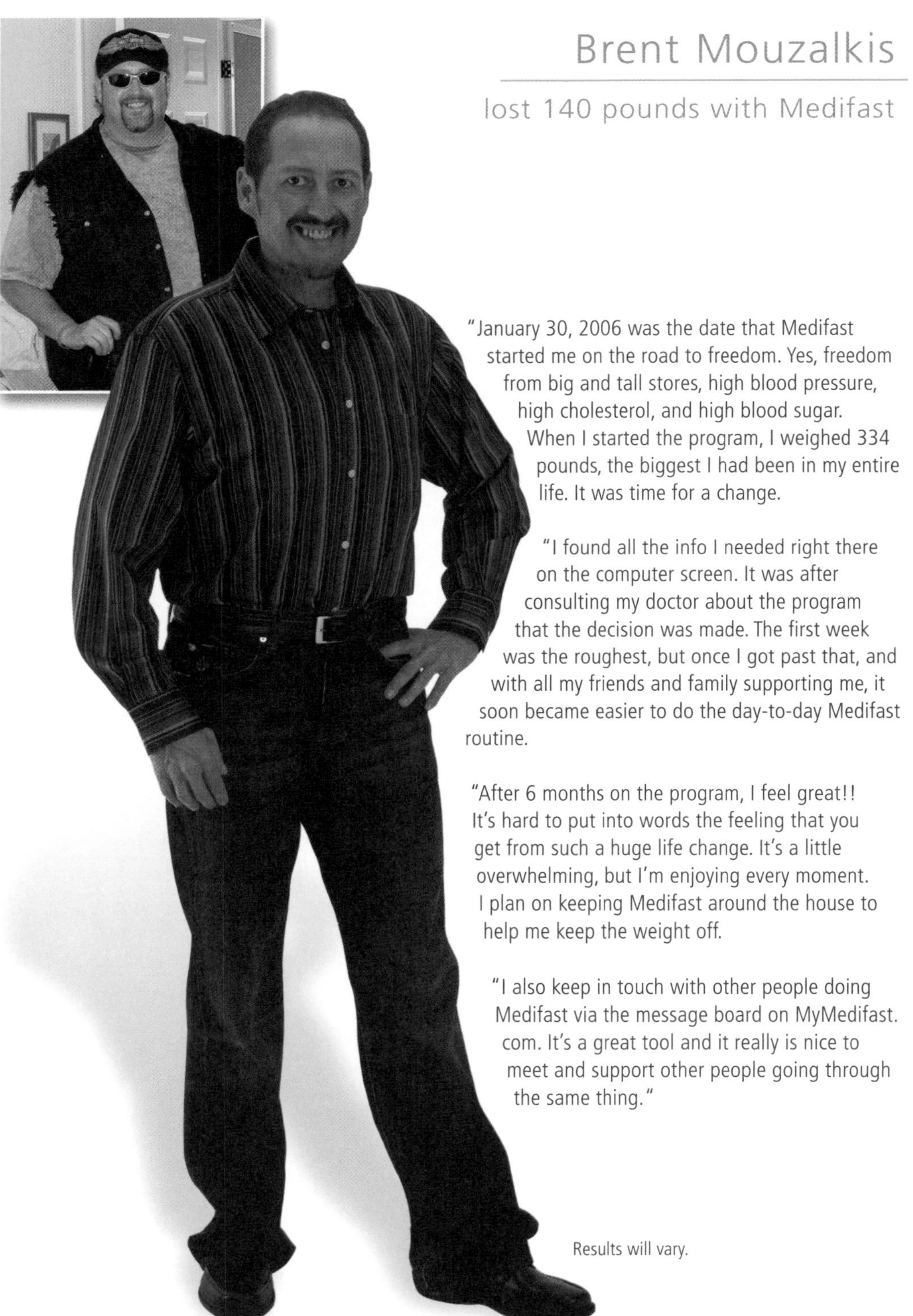

Brent Mouzalkis

lost 140 pounds with Medifast

"January 30, 2006 was the date that Medifast started me on the road to freedom. Yes, freedom from big and tall stores, high blood pressure, high cholesterol, and high blood sugar. When I started the program, I weighed 334 pounds, the biggest I had been in my entire life. It was time for a change.

"I found all the info I needed right there on the computer screen. It was after consulting my doctor about the program that the decision was made. The first week was the roughest, but once I got past that, and with all my friends and family supporting me, it soon became easier to do the day-to-day Medifast routine.

"After 6 months on the program, I feel great!! It's hard to put into words the feeling that you get from such a huge life change. It's a little overwhelming, but I'm enjoying every moment. I plan on keeping Medifast around the house to help me keep the weight off.

"I also keep in touch with other people doing Medifast via the message board on MyMedifast.com. It's a great tool and it really is nice to meet and support other people going through the same thing."

Results will vary.

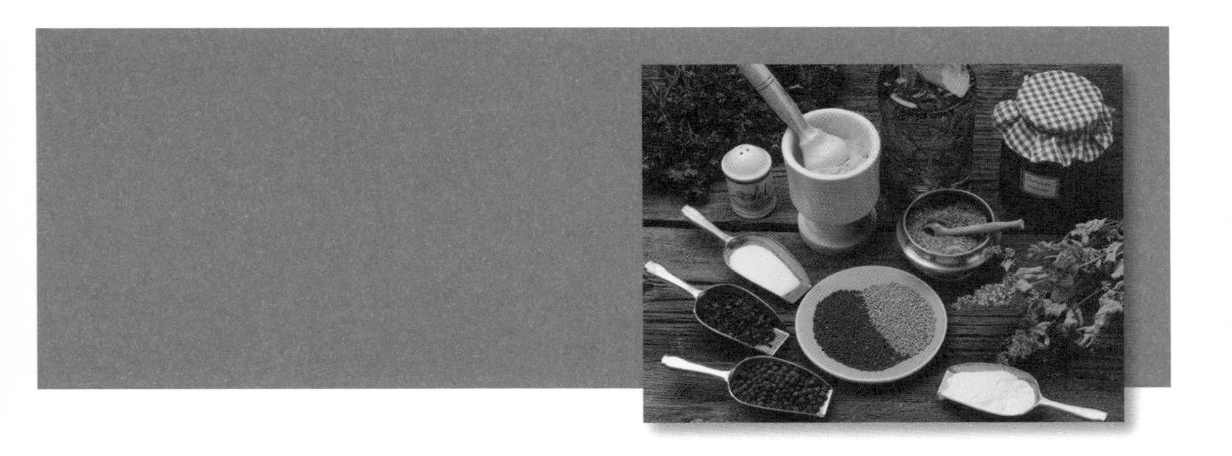

12 Nutritionally enhanced foods for health

"Let food be your medicine."
~Hippocrates

One of the unique features that sets Medifast apart from the rest is that Medifast foods have been nutritionally enhanced to support both the weight loss and health needs of men and women.

This chapter will provide you with detailed information about health conditions that affect both overweight men and overweight women. It will focus on three specific health conditions, diabetes, coronary heart disease, and arthritis. It details how Medifast foods have been nutritionally balanced to help improve the health of individuals suffering from these conditions, in addition to aiding these people in their weight control efforts.

There are at least three ways Medifast Meals can improve the health of overweight men and women:

> **Through weight loss.** Losing just five to 10 percent of your body weight may decrease your risk of heart disease, diabetes, certain cancers, and other conditions—not to mention the cost savings on medications used to control high blood pressure and diabetes, and the discomfort, complications, and doctor bills that having such conditions bring.

Through the use of soy protein. Not only is soy protein a high quality protein, it is thought to play both a preventive and a therapeutic role in cardiovascular disease, cancer, and osteoporosis, as well as alleviate the symptoms of menopause. Many Medifast Meals contain enough soy protein to have earned the FDA health claim "heart healthy."

Through the addition of health-enhancing ingredients shown to aid specific health conditions.

Medifast has created three lines of nutritionally enhanced meals to target these conditions, Medifast Plus for Diabetics, Medifast Plus for Coronary Health, and Medifast Plus for Joint Health. The following table provides an overview of these products. Highlighted in the table are the main health-promoting ingredients used in the creation of each meal type.

Medifast Plus for Diabetics

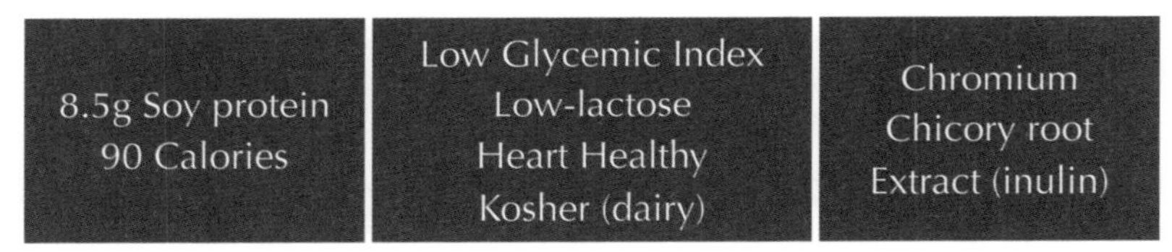

8.5g Soy protein 90 Calories	Low Glycemic Index Low-lactose Heart Healthy Kosher (dairy)	Chromium Chicory root Extract (inulin)

Medifast Plus for Coronary Health

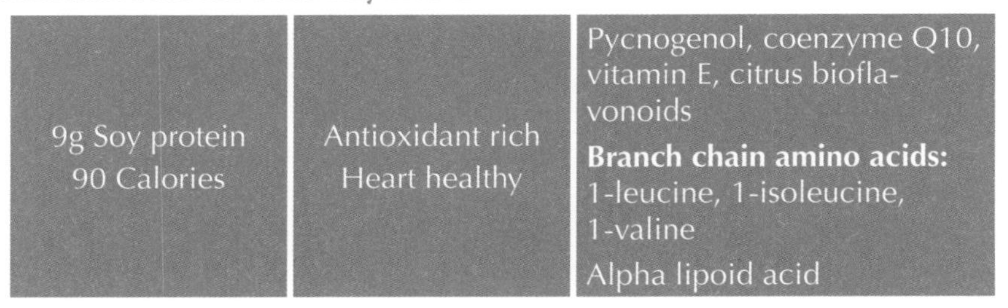

9g Soy protein 90 Calories	Antioxidant rich Heart healthy	Pycnogenol, coenzyme Q10, vitamin E, citrus bioflavonoids **Branch chain amino acids:** 1-leucine, 1-isoleucine, 1-valine Alpha lipoid acid

Medifast Plus for Joint Health

9g Soy protein 90 Calories	Joint-supporting Diabetic-friendly Heart healthy	Glucasamine Chondroitin (shark cartilidge) Calcium and vitamin D Chicory root extract Chromium

NOTE: The soy protein and calorie figures listed in the table are single-meal totals (e.g., a shake or a bar).

If you are already suffering from diabetes, coronary heart disease, or arthritis, then you are likely familiar with general health information about each condition (and the specific signs/symptoms to watch out for). For education and awareness purposes, we have provided general information about each condition, and how to recognize condition-specific signs and symptoms. Of course, please consult with your primary health care provider about specific diagnoses and treatments for these conditions.

Diabetes

Diabetes is a chronic health condition characterized by high blood glucose (sugar) levels. Normally, your blood always has some glucose in it because your body turns the foods you eat into glucose for energy. Insulin is released from the pancreas to help transport this energy to the cells. If your body doesn't make enough insulin or if the insulin doesn't work the way it should, glucose can't get into your cells, so it stays in your bloodstream. Your blood glucose level then gets too high, resulting in diabetes.

Diabetes can be harmful when blood sugar levels run high for extended periods of time. It can potentially damage vital organs like your eyes, kidneys, heart, and blood vessels. In the United States, diabetes (and its complications) is currently the third leading cause of death. Approximately 75 percent of people with diabetes die from some form of heart or blood vessel disease.

There are two main types of diabetes. Type 1 diabetes (insulin-dependent diabetes) is usually first diagnosed in children, teenagers, or young adults. It results when the beta cells of the pancreas no longer make insulin (the body's own immune system attacks and destroys the beta cells). Treatment for type 1 diabetes includes daily (or more frequent) insulin injections or use of an insulin pump.

Type 2 diabetes (non-insulin-dependent diabetes) is the most common form of diabetes. People can develop type 2 diabetes at any age—even during childhood. In type 2 diabetes, the pancreas does not make enough insulin and the fat, muscle, or liver cells do not use it properly. Being overweight can increase the chance of developing type 2 diabetes. For many, treatment includes diabetes medications (sometimes even insulin), making wise food choices, exercising regularly, taking a daily aspirin, and controlling blood pressure and cholesterol.

The connection between weight loss and diabetes

The bad news is that overweight people are far more likely than lean individuals to develop type 2 diabetes. According to the American Obesity Association, as many as 90 percent of individuals with diabetes are either overweight or obese. The good news is that losing weight can help control the signs and symptoms of type 2 diabetes. In fact, losing just five percent of your body weight may be enough to get high blood sugar levels under control, and may even reduce the need for medication.

Medifast Plus for Diabetics

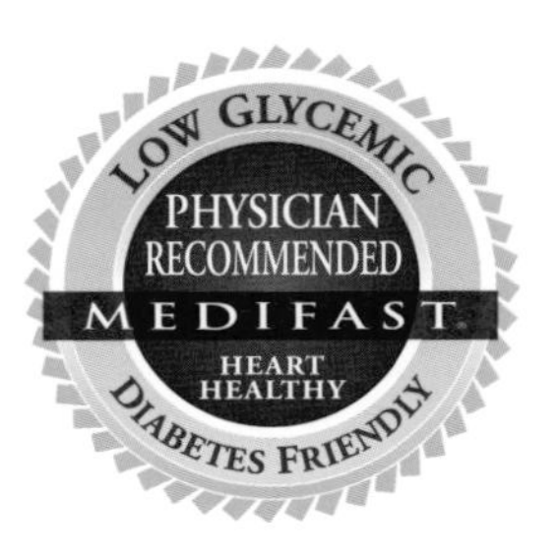

Medifast Plus for Diabetics Shakes have been specially formulated to meet the health and weight loss needs of people with diabetes. These meals are soy-based, portion-controlled, and nutritionally enhanced. Moreover, they rank low on the glycemic index (GI) scale, so they aid in the control of blood sugar levels.

Please note that all Medifast products are suitable for people with type 2 diabetes. It is essential that you see your physician or diabetes specialist prior to starting and during your Medifast program to discuss blood sugar monitoring, potassium monitoring, oral diabetes agents, appropriate calorie levels, and potential adjustments to your medications.

Medifast Plus for Diabetics has been clinically studied and proven to work. Compared to a diet based on recommendations of the American Diabetes Association (ADA), Medifast significantly reduced body weight and blood sugar levels among overweight and obese individuals with type 2 diabetes. Dieters on Medifast lost twice as much weight after 34 weeks; an average of 16 pounds, compared to only eight pounds on the ADA diet. The weight loss on Medifast resulted in significant reductions in blood glucose and insulin levels compared to pre-treatment values. Perhaps more important, significantly more individuals in the Medifast group were able to reduce their use of diabetes medications compared to those in the ADA diet group. After 86-weeks, 36 percent of subjects on Medifast were off of their blood sugar medications entirely.

Since Medifast Plus for Diabetics Shakes have a low glycemic index (GI), they do not cause spikes in blood sugar levels. Containing less than six grams of sugar per serving and nine grams total carbohydrates per serving, Medifast Plus for Diabetics Shakes have been certified LOW GLYCEMIC by the Glycemic Research Institute, and therefore are authorized to use the Glycemic Research

Institute's Seal of Approval. Low GI foods break down slowly, so glucose is gradually released into the blood stream, allowing blood glucose to rise slowly. High GI foods break down quickly during digestion, are rapidly released into the bloodstream, and raise blood glucose rapidly.

- Low GI foods are satiating (keep you feeling full longer) because they are more filling than high GI foods. This may be why dieters on Medifast stick to the program better. Compliance data shows that almost twice as many people in the study who were on Medifast completed the weight loss portion of their diet compared to those following the diet modeled on recommendations of the American Diabetes Association.
- Many contain soy protein. Soy protein has been shown to improve markers of diabetic kidney disease (protein in the urine) in type 2 diabetes patients. Switching from animal-based protein (casein) to soy protein has been shown to decrease unwanted proteins in the urine.[46]
- Medifast Plus for Diabetics foods are formulated with chicory root extract (inulin) which may stimulate gastrointestinal proteins that decrease appetite, leading to reductions in body weight, glucose, and insulin levels.
- Medifast Plus for Diabetics foods contain chromium, which plays an integral role in carbohydrate metabolism by helping insulin to do its job. Studies have shown that for people with diabetes, chromium supplementation improves blood sugar, insulin, and hemoglobin A1c levels (a measure of blood sugar control over the previous few months).

Frequently asked questions (FAQs) about Medifast Plus for Diabetics

How do I use Medifast Plus for Diabetics for weight loss?

Medifast recommends that you consult with your primary care provider or diabetes specialist before beginning a program using Medifast Plus for Diabetics. You should discuss with your healthcare provider blood sugar monitoring, and possibly changing doses of any oral diabetes agents and insulin you may be taking before starting the program. We suggest using Medifast Plus for Diabetics as a program that includes 5 Medifast Meals and 1 Lean & Green Meal per day (the Lean & Green Meal on this program should include a salad and a vegetable).

Should I continue my oral diabetes medication(s)?

Medifast Meals are likely to provide a much lower level of calories and carbohydrates than your current diet, so it is prudent to check your blood sugar at least two to three times daily, especially at the beginning of the Medifast Program. If your blood sugar levels fall below the range specified by your doctor, you should seek his advice.

What if I'm on insulin?

Prior to beginning the program, Medifast recommends that you consult with your primary care provider about your current insulin dosage. Blood sugar testing should be performed several times throughout the day. As your blood sugar level drops, continue consulting with your doctor about changes in your insulin requirements.

Coronary heart disease

Coronary heart disease occurs when the inside walls of the coronary arteries become narrowed or clogged with plaque deposits. The narrowing or clogging of arteries reduces the flow of oxygen- and nutrient-rich blood to the heart. It often occurs in a person who has high levels of cholesterol and/or triglycerides, which are fat-like substances in the blood. Cholesterol and triglycerides flowing in the blood, build up on the walls of the arteries. The build-up of plaque thickens the arteries and can slow (or totally block) the circulation of blood, as occurs in the case of a heart attack and some forms of stroke.

Connection between weight loss and coronary health

The higher the level of cholesterol in the bloodstream, the greater the possibility that plaque will be deposited on the walls of arteries. Overweight and obesity increase the risk of developing high blood cholesterol as well as high blood pressure, both of which increase the chance of developing coronary heart disease. The risk is even greater if you add cigarette smoking to the mix. Losing just five to 10 percent of your body weight may improve high blood pressure and high cholesterol, thus reducing your risk of coronary artery disease. Weight loss with Medifast is appropriate for individuals with coronary heart disease, assuming that your primary care provider says there are no contraindications to its use.

Risk factors for cardiovascular disease

The American Heart Association has identified several risk factors for heart disease. Some of them can be modified, treated, or controlled—some of them cannot. A general rule of thumb is that the more risk factors you have, the greater your chance of developing heart disease.

Major risk factors that can NOT be changed:

Advancing age

Over 83 percent of people who die of cardiovascular disease are 65 or older.

Gender

Men have a greater risk of heart attack than women do, and they generally have heart attacks earlier in life.

Heredity (including race)

Children of parents with cardiovascular disease are more likely to develop it themselves. African-Americans, Latinos, Native Americans, Hawaiians, and some Asian Americans are at higher risk. This is partly related to higher rates of obesity and type 2 diabetes in these populations.

Major risk factors that CAN be changed:

Tobacco smoke

People who smoke are two to four times more likely than nonsmokers to develop cardiovascular disease. Cigar or pipe smokers seem to have a higher risk of death from coronary artery disease (and possibly stroke) but their risk is not as great as cigarette smokers' risk. Even for non-smokers, exposure to other people's smoke (second-hand smoke) increases the risk of cardiovascular disease.

High blood cholesterol

As blood cholesterol rises, so does the risk of cardiovascular disease.

High blood pressure

High blood pressure increases how hard the heart has to work. The heart is a muscle, so the harder it has to work, the thicker and stiffer it becomes. While thicker biceps and triceps may be desirable, a thicker heart muscle is not.

Physical inactivity

Regular, moderate-to-vigorous physical activity helps prevent cardiovascular disease.

Obesity/overweight

People who have excess body fat (especially around the waist) are more likely to develop heart disease and stroke, even in the absence of other risk factors. Excess weight increases the heart's workload. It also raises blood pressure, blood cholesterol, and triglyceride levels, and lowers the level of HDL (good) cholesterol. It also increases the risk of developing type 2 diabetes.

Diabetes

Diabetes seriously increases your risk of heart attack and stroke, particularly if blood sugar is poorly controlled. About three-quarters of people with diabetes die from some form of heart or blood vessel disease.

Stress

Individual responses to stress may be a contributing factor. When people are stressed, they may overeat, start smoking, or smoke more than they otherwise would.

Alcohol

Drinking too much alcohol (more than two servings a day) can raise blood pressure, cause heart failure, or lead to stroke. One drink is defined as:

- 1-½ fluid ounces of 80-proof spirits (such as bourbon, Scotch, vodka, gin, etc.)
- 1 fluid ounce of 100-proof spirits
- 4 fluid ounces of wine
- 12 fluid ounces of beer

How can I assess my risk of developing heart disease?

The National Heart, Lung, and Blood Institute (NHLBI) launched the National Cholesterol Education Program (NCEP) with the goal of reducing illness and death from coronary heart disease (CHD) in the United States. The NHLBI has developed a risk assessment tool that you can use to determine your risk of developing heart disease over the next 10 years.

Here is what the risk assessment tool looks like. You can gather the information necessary to calculate your risk, and then do so online at the following web address: http:hp2010.nhlbihin.net/atpiii/calculator.asp?usertype=pub

Signs and symptoms of coronary heart disease include:

- shortness of breath
- cold sweat
- nausea
- light-headedness
- chest pain (burning, tightness, heaviness, pain, pressure, or squeezing usually in your chest but sometimes also in the arms, neck, or jaws)
- no symptoms at all

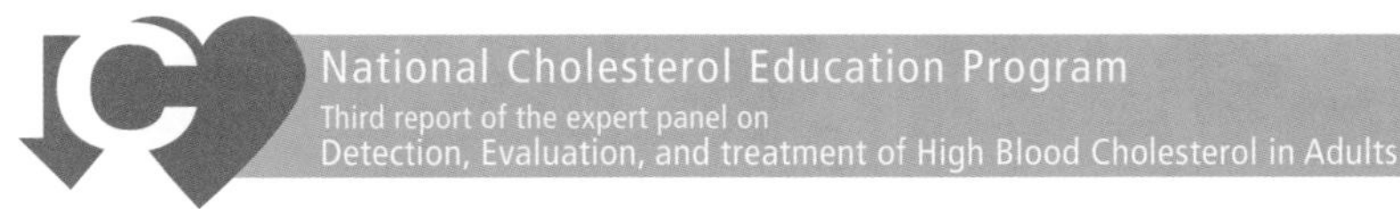

Risk Assessment Tool for Estimating Your 10-year Risk of having a heart attack

The risk assessment tool below uses information from the Framingham Heart Study to predict a person's chance of having a heart attack in the next 10 years. This tool is designed for adults age 20 and older who do not have heart disease or diabetes. To find your risk score, enter your information in the form below.

Age:	______ years
Gender:	❑ male ❑ female
Total Cholesterol:	______ mg/dL
HDL Cholesterol:	______ mg/dL
Smoker:	❑ no ❑ yes
Systolic Blood Pressure:	______ mm/Hg
Are you currently on any medication to treat high blood pressure?	❑ no ❑ yes

Total Cholesterol – Total cholesterol is the sum of all the cholesterol in your blood. The higher your total cholesterol, the greater your risk for heart disease. Here are the total values that matter to you:

Less than 200 mg/dL: "Desirable" level that puts you at lower risk for heart disease. A cholesterol level of 200 mg/dL or greater increases your risk.

200 to 239 mg/dL: "Borderline-high"

240 mg/dL and above: "High" blood cholesterol. A person with this level has more than twice the risk of heart disease compared to someone whose cholesterol is below 200 mg/dL.

HDL Cholesterol – High-density lipoproteins (HDL) is the "good" cholesterol. HDL carry cholesterol in the blood from other parts of the body back to the liver, which leads to its removal from the body. So HDL help keep cholesterol from building up in the walls of the arteries. Here are the HDL-cholesterol levels that matter to you.

Less than 40 mg/dL: A major risk factor for heart disease.

40 to 59 mg/dL: The higher your HDL, the better.

60 mg/dL: and above. An HDL of 60 mg/dL and above is considered protective against heart disease.

Smoker – Select "yes" if you have smoked any cigarettes in the past month.

Systolic blood pressure – Systolic blood pressure is the first number of your blood pressure reading. For example, if your reading is 120/80 (120 over 80), your systolic blood pressure is 120.

The severity of symptoms varies widely. Your symptoms may become more severe as your coronary arteries become narrower or clogged with cholesterol plaques.

Medifast Plus for Coronary Health

Medifast Plus for Coronary Health consists of foods that have been nutritionally enhanced to produce weight loss, while at the same time protect against heart disease. Formulated with the highest quality nutrients, vitamins and minerals, Medifast Plus for Coronary Health provides a natural defense against heart disease.

Below are the ingredients found in Medifast Plus for Coronary Health Shakes that may help protect against coronary disease.

Soy protein

Dozens of controlled clinical studies have shown that foods rich in soy protein are good for coronary health. Soy protein has been shown to lower levels of total cholesterol, triglycerides, and low-density lipoprotein (LDL, or bad cholesterol), without affecting the amount of high-density lipoprotein (HDL, or good cholesterol). According to the Food and Drug Administration (FDA), diets with four daily servings of soy (25 g/day) can reduce levels of LDLs by as much as 10 percent. The FDA allows the health claim "heart healthy" to be placed on labels of foods that may help lower heart disease risk. To qualify for the heart healthy claim, foods must:

- Contain 6.25 grams of soy protein per serving
- Be low-fat (less than 3 grams)
- Be low in saturated fats (less than 1 gram)
- Be low-cholesterol (less than 20 milligrams)
- Have a sodium value of less than 480 milligrams for individual foods, less than 720 milligrams if considered a main dish, and less than 960 milligrams if considered a meal.

Specific components of soy, such as soluble fiber and antioxidants may be beneficial to heart health.

Soluble fiber

Soybeans contain soluble fiber, which may benefit heart disease by interfering with the absorption and metabolism of cholesterol. In the gut, fiber binds with fatty acids and excretes them through the gastrointestinal

(GI) tract. Fiber has been shown to reduce both total cholesterol and LDL cholesterol.

Isoflavone antioxidants

Genistein and Diadzein are two isoflavones that protect the heart. They boost the activity of LDL receptors which remove LDL cholesterol from the bloodstream, and deliver it to the liver where it is broken down and excreted from the body. They also protect the heart by reducing blood clots that can lead to heart attacks, and may inhibit the growth of cells that form plaque inside.

Other cardioprotective nutrients in soy

Soybeans are also a good source of lecithin and vitamin E. Lecithin and vitamin E are natural antioxidants that help prevent the oxidation of LDL cholesterol.

Antioxidants (other than those found in soy)

Medifast Plus for Coronary Health meals are nutritionally enhanced with certain antioxidants known to be heart healthy as well. These meals are fortified with antioxidant vitamins (like E and C), and beta-carotene (known to be part of the body's natural defense system). Beta-carotene may also help protect against cardiovascular disease. Medifast Plus for Coronary Health also includes antioxidants that benefit heart health like coenzyme Q10, citrus bioflavonoids, pycnogenol, and alpha lipoic acid. Let's take a closer look at them.

Coenzyme Q10

Coenzyme Q10 (CoQ10), or ubiquinone, is a vitamin-like substance found in small amounts in a wide variety of foods. CoQ10 is known to be highly concentrated in heart muscle cells. This nutrient has been shown to reduce plaque build-up in arteries and reduce the occurrence of plaque rupture, both of which can lead to heart attacks.

Individuals who have low amounts of CoQ10 are more likely to have heart problems like congestive heart failure (from a wide variety of causes). The severity of heart failure has been associated with the severity of CoQ10 deficiency. There have been numerous international studies evaluating CoQ10 in heart disease and congestive heart failure, and all have found CoQ10 to be effective and safe.

Citrus bioflavonoids and pycnogenol

Citrus pycnogenol (revenol) and bioflavinoids are part of a group of beneficial plant substances with antioxidant properties known as polyphenols.

Pycnogenol is found in the bark of pine trees, and citrus bioflavonoids are found in citrus fruits (e.g., lemons and oranges). Both are heart-protective antioxidants that have been linked to lower levels of cardiovascular disease. Pycnogenol has also been shown to reduce the clumping of platelets in individuals who smoke (similar to aspirin).

Alpha lipoic acid

Alpha Lipoic Acid is an antioxidant that quenches free radicals and by doing so gets rid of harmful oxidants that damage cells and cause inflammation, especially to the heart. It may also play an important role in the body's network of antioxidants by extending the metabolic lifespan of other antioxidants like vitamin C, glutathione, and coenzyme Q10 (and indirectly by renewing vitamin E).

Amino acids (the good and the bad)

The good

The branched chain amino acids (BCAAs) leucine, isoleucine, and valine, are amino acids associated with coronary health benefits. These essential amino acids are found mostly in muscle tissue and help to boost the muscle-building process. Since it is a muscle, the heart may also benefit from BCAAs. When there is an increased need for BCAAs (as in the case of a heart attack), BCAAs can provide an alternate energy substrate for the heart.

Carnitine is another heart-healthy amino acid. It has been found to lower serum cholesterol and triglyceride levels, build muscle tissue, and increase stamina. A low level of carnitine may cause muscle weakness, confusion, or chest pain. A deficiency can also lead to a higher level of fat (triglycerides) in your bloodstream.

The bad

Many of you may have heard of the amino acid "homocysteine." High levels of homocysteine are associated with cardiovascular disease, strokes, and peripheral vascular disease (fatty deposits in peripheral arteries). Evidence shows that when blood levels of folic acid are low, homocysteine levels are higher; elevating the risk of coronary heart disease and stroke. Folic acid (and other B vitamins) help reduce homocysteine levels by breaking it down in the body. It is often recommended that individuals with high homocysteine levels, or those at risk of having high levels (e.g., family history), take folic acid. That is why Medifast Plus for Coronary Health is fortified with folic acid and other B vitamins (especially B-6 and B-12).

Chicory root extract (Inulin)

One other notable ingredient in Medifast Plus for Coronary Health is chicory root extract. Diabetes greatly increases the risk of heart disease. Chicory root extract can help improve diabetes by reducing body weight and blood sugar levels; thereby helping to reduce the risk of heart disease.

FAQs about Medifast Plus for Coronary Health

How do I use Medifast Plus for Coronary Health?

Medifast Plus for Coronary Health meals can be used one to three times a day as part of your Medifast Program. They can also be used outside of the Medifast Program as a snack or occasional meal replacement for general health.

Is Medifast Plus for Coronary Health safe to take with my medications?

Do not stop taking your medication(s) while using Medifast Plus for Coronary Health unless directed to do so by your health care provider. Unless your primary health care provider has told you otherwise, Medifast Plus for Coronary Health may be taken with your medications.

Joint health/arthritis

According to the National Arthritis Foundation, arthritis affects nearly one out of every six Americans, making it one of the most common medical conditions in the United States. In addition, arthritis is the leading cause of disability, limiting the daily activities of more than seven million Americans. Osteoarthritis (OA) is the most common form of arthritis, and is prevalent in over 80 percent of adults aged 55 and older. OA is a joint condition caused by "wear and tear" on the joint cartilage, the tissue that cushions bones where they meet.

The connection between weight loss, joint health, and OA

Being overweight is associated with an increased risk of osteoarthritis. According to data from the first National Health and Nutrition Examination Survey (NHANES I), overweight and obese women had nearly four times the risk of knee OA as compared with non-obese women. Obese men had a nearly five times greater risk. Weight loss has been shown to reduce the risk of OA of the knees. According to the American Obesity Association, a modest weight loss of

10 to 15 pounds may relieve the symptoms of arthritis.

Permanent weight control can decrease the wear and tear on your joints, delay the progression of arthritis, and decrease the risk of developing surgical complications (should surgery ever be needed to relieve arthritis symptoms).

Signs and Symptoms of OA:

- Recurring joint pain (usually affecting knees, hips, hands, cervical and lumbar spine, and the smallest joints on fingers)
- Stiffness (frequent but brief in the morning and after inactivity)
- Inflammation (warmth/tenderness)
- Swelling in one or more joints

Medifast Plus for Joint Health

To help relieve the symptoms of arthritis, many people use anti-inflammatory and pain-relieving medications. These medications may relieve symptoms of OA, but they do not prevent cartilage from deteriorating and may actually have harmful effects when taken for prolonged periods of time. The use of aspirin or aspirin-like nonsteroidal anti-inflammatory agents is the number one cause of upper gastrointestinal ulcers and bleeding. Medifast Plus for Joint Health Shakes are a safe and effective way to improve joint health without the worry of such side effects. Below are the ingredients found in these shakes that may help to maximize joint health.

Glucosamine sulfate/chondroitin sulfate

Supplements containing glucosamine sulfate and chondroitin sulfate (shark cartilage) have been shown to be safe and effective, and may aid in repairing joint health. In fact, results of the NIH-funded Glucosamine Arthritis Intervention Trial (GAIT), found that glucosamine/chondroitin was as effective (if not more effective) than the popular arthritis drug Celebrex in treating moderate to severe arthritic pain.

Chondroitin sulfate may help repair the structure and function of cartilage. Glucosamine may improve joint elasticity, increase range of motion, and may slow or even reverse joint damage. Solid scientific research has shown that glucosamine is effective for:

- Reducing joint pain/anti-inflammatory actions
- Increasing lubrication of the joint
- Inhibiting the break down of cartilage
- Stimulating repair of the cartilage matrix

Soy protein

Soy has anti-inflammatory properties that may improve the symptoms of OA. In addition to reducing pain and inflammation, it has been shown to improve knee range of motion and improve the condition of cartilage tissue.

Vitamins and minerals

Medifast Plus for Joint Health also contains a special mix of vitamins and minerals known to be good for your bones and joints. Calcium and vitamin D help to build and maintain healthy bones and joints. Vitamin C is necessary for collagen formation, a main component of bones and cartilage that gives them form and substance.

Chicory root extract

There is some evidence that chicory root extract may have anti-inflammatory properties that would be useful in OA. Chicory root extract may decrease inflammation by inhibiting cyclooxygenase-2 (COX-2) protein.[47] Therefore, it may offer a safer alternative to the newest line of arthritis drugs known as COX-2 inhibitors (e.g., Celebrex) that improve pain and reduce inflammation.

FAQs about Medifast Plus for Joint Health

Who should use Medifast Plus for Joint Health?

Medifast Plus for Joint Health is recommended for individuals over the age of 18 who suffer with painful joints due to arthritis and/or injury.

How do I use Medifast Plus for Joint Health?

For optimal joint health, Medifast Plus for Joint Health should be taken one to three times a day as part of your Medifast Program. It can also be used outside of a Medifast Program as a snack or occasional meal replacement.

Medifast and other health conditions

Men and women who lose weight on Medifast, experience health benefits for diabetes, coronary disease, and arthritis—and for other conditions as well. The soy in Medifast may help prevent certain kinds of cancer. The weight loss you can achieve from following the Medifast program may also improve the symptoms associated with sleep apnea, reduce fatigue, and enhance psychological health. The psychological benefits of losing weight with Medifast can be enormous.

Permanent weight control can provide impressive emotional benefits in both mood and overall quality of life.

Medifast weight control in children and adolescents

The benefits of Medifast are not limited to just adults. Youth who are struggling with their weight can also reap the benefits of Medifast. Obesity statistics show that over the past 25 years, obesity rates among adolescents (ages 12 to 19) have doubled, and among children (ages 6 to 11) have quadrupled. As a result, many of the health problems associated with overweight adults like diabetes, high cholesterol, and high blood pressure are now being seen in our youth. Furthermore, childhood obesity has emotional consequences, with many kids suffering from psychological distress, low self-esteem, and poor body image.

Because children who are overweight or obese are likely to become overweight or obese adults, the best time to address the problem is now. If you are wondering if your child is overweight or obese, it is important to talk with your child's doctor. The doctor will use the child's height and weight to determine if they have a weight problem based on the following criteria: Overweight in children means having a BMI at or above the 85th percentile. The 85th percentile corresponds to a BMI of 25 kg/m2. Obesity in children means having a BMI at or over the 95th percentile. The 95th percentile corresponds to a BMI of 30 kg/m2.

According to the American Obesity Association (AOA), 30 percent of children (ages 6 to 11) and adolescents (ages 12 to 19) are overweight, and 15 percent of both children and adolescents are considered obese. Genetic predisposition may play a role in the development of kids being overweight, especially if parents and/or siblings are overweight. However, poor dietary habits and physical inactivity are the main reasons for the obesity epidemic seen in youth today.

For some youth, simply watching their diet more closely and increasing their physical activity levels is enough to gain control of their weight. For many, however, it is not enough. For this group of youths, there is without a doubt a need for more potent interventions. Some of these more potent interventions, however, have included some fairly drastic measures. For instance, more youth than ever before are being prescribed weight-loss medications and having obesity surgery, with the justification that the benefits of these more extreme measures outweigh the health risks of doing nothing at all. But do we really want to go there? Do we really want our kids undergoing major abdominal surgery to control their weight problems? I think most of us, especially parents, would opt for a less risky intervention.

The concept of structured meals or meal replacements is potent intervention, and has fewer risks than weight-loss medications or gastric bypass surgery. Meal replacements have been shown to safely cause weight loss in children and are probably under-appreciated as a treatment resource. Recognizing the need for a safe, yet potent intervention, Medifast has tested its line of nutritionally enhanced foods in kids as young as eight years old. This study found that youth on Medifast safely lost weight when following the 5 & 1 Plan.

Moreover, to meet the nutritional needs of the youth, Medifast Meals are fortified with all the vitamins and minerals growing children and adolescents need.

The health benefits of weight loss (both physical and psychological) are immense. Medifast's nutritionally enhanced meals can help both adults and youth achieve their weight-loss goals, and at the same time improve their physical health and emotional well-being. To learn more about how Medifast can meet the gender-specific weight loss and health needs of women and men, please refer to chapters 10 and 11, respectively.

Mary Jane Medlock

lost 170 pounds with Medifast

"I have spent over $20,000 on weight-loss products, programs, and pills with little or no success. Finally, I found the Medifast Program. I had extraordinary results.

"I lost over 170 pounds, went from a size 56 to an 8, and have not gained one pound back.

"For a person that was used to jumping from one diet to another, I have not been on any other program since the year 2001. That is truly a miracle in itself.

"With Medifast, I didn't have to count calories, carbs, fat grams, or mess with portion sizes. This program is literally GOOF-PROOF!!

"For years, I felt like a failure with no hope, but all I needed was Medifast, which gave me rapid, continuous weight loss and tremendous energy.

"No pills, no stomach surgery, NO KIDDING!!.

"I hope that my story inspires others because I now live my life with complete passion and fulfillment. If I can do it, so can you."

Results will vary.

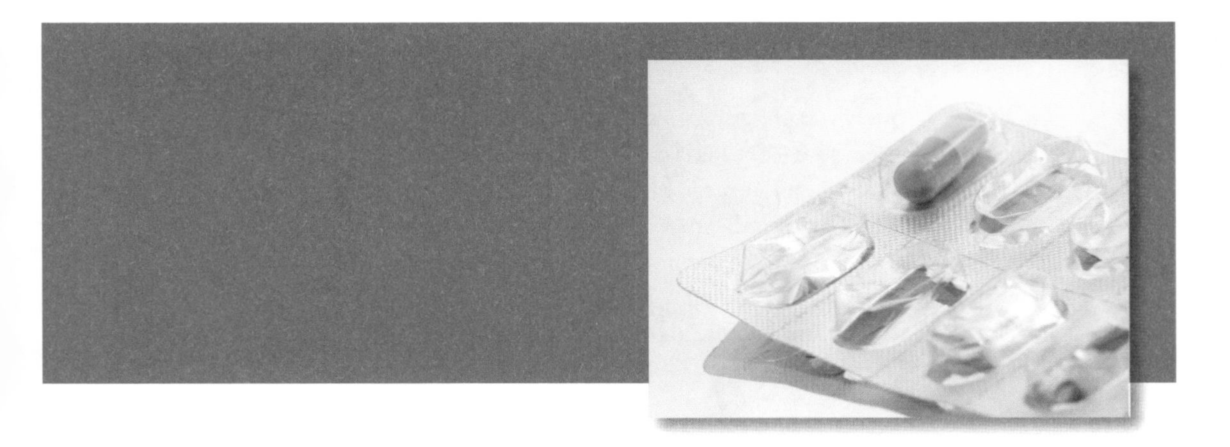

13 Weight-loss medications and obesity surgery

Many of you may be curious about other options available for aiding weight-loss efforts. You may have thought about taking appetite suppressants or have even considered surgery for weight reduction. In order for you to make informed decisions about these more extreme measures of weight control, this chapter will provide you with up-to-date information about weight-loss medications and surgical options for obesity. The goal of this chapter, however, is not to advocate these more extreme measures for controlling weight. For most people, the Medifast Program alone naturally suppresses appetite and eliminates hunger (without requiring other therapies). The goal of this chapter is to inform you about weight-loss medications and surgical options for obesity so you can determine whether the benefits of such approaches are worth the risks, especially when you can potentially achieve the same weight loss with Medifast alone (with far less risk). Finally, for those who have opted for medication and/or surgery, this chapter also shows you that Medifast can be safely used to augment these other therapies.

Please understand in reading this chapter that general information is provided that may not apply to you. You must consult with your doctor to determine whether you are a candidate for weight-loss medications or obesity surgery.

Generally, before either weight-loss medications or surgery are permitted, a behavioral approach to weight loss (diet and exercise) must be tried for at least six months. If diet and exercise have failed to help you achieve your weight-loss goals after six months, medications and surgery become potential options. These options, however, are not for everyone. There are strict criteria that you must meet to be considered a candidate for either of these forms of treatment. They should also be considered add-ons to dietary and behavioral modifications, not treatments that are sufficient in and of themselves.

Weight-loss medications

Before getting into details about the medications available to treat obesity, you might want to know whether or not you are a candidate for taking such drugs. The FDA has specific criteria that individuals must meet in order to be prescribed weight-loss medications as part of their weight-loss plan. FDA recommendations are that you have a BMI of:

27 kg/m² plus serious obesity-related health conditions
(e.g., high blood pressure, high cholesterol, type 2 diabetes)

OR

30 kg/m² without obesity-related health conditions

A close look at weight-loss medications

Now that you know whether or not you would meet the criteria to be prescribed weight-loss medications, let's take a closer look at what is available. Despite having spent many millions of dollars in research and development of agents for the treatment of obesity, the current arsenal of FDA approved anti-obesity agents is actually quite slim. As of this writing, there are only two FDA approved medications for safe and effective long-term (one to two years) treatment: orlistat (Xenical) and sibutramine (Meridia). There are, however, four other anti-obesity agents that are approved for the short-term (<12 weeks) treatment of obesity: benzphetamine, phendimetrazine, phentermine and diethylpropion. Of this class of agents, phentermine is probably the most widely known and prescribed, and so will be the agent discussed in further detail. Also briefly described will be medications that are not FDA approved for the treatment of obesity, but have been associated with reductions in appetite and body weight. And finally, information will be provided about a promising new weight-loss agent on the horizon, rimonabant (Accomplia). The following table provides a brief description of weight-loss agents that will be covered in this chapter:

FDA-approved for weight control appetite suppressants

Medication	Description
Sibutramine (Meridia)	• Norepinephrine and serotonin re-uptake inhibitor; approved for long-term treatment of obesity combined with low-calorie diet • Reduces appetite and increases thermogenesis (turns fat into heat and energy).
Phentermine (Ionamin, Adipex-P, fastin)	• Sympathomimetic amine that stimulates the release of nor-epinephrine and dopamine • Approved for short-term weight loss with low-calorie diet. Its similar structure to amphetamine may lead to the development of dependence and tolerance
Orlistat (Xenical) Lipase inhibitor	• Prevents the digestion and absorption of dietary fat (approximately 30%), including fat-soluble vitamins

Other (not FDA-approved for weight control)

Medication	Description
Fluoxetine (Prozac)	• Serotonin re-uptake inhibitor (SSRI) approved for the treatment of depression. Investigated as a weight-loss agent and found to have appetite suppressant/weight-loss effect for about six months
Bupropion SR (Wellbutrin, Zyban)	• Nonrepinephrine and dopamine re-uptake inhibitor used for depression and smoking cessation, associated with reduced appetite and weight loss
Zonisamide (Zonegran)	• Approved for treatment of partial (focal) seizures in adults with epilepsy and shown to reduce appetite.
Topiramate (Topamax)	• Anti-convulsant for treatment of refractory seizures in combination with other anti-seizure medications: used in treatment of mood disorders where observed to reduce weight gain associated with anti-depressant therapy

FDA-approved for weight control (long term)

Sibutramine (Meridia)

Sibutramine is a serotonin and norepinephrine re-uptake inhibitor. It is similar to some commonly used anti-depressants, like Prozac. It works to decrease appetite by blocking the re-uptake of neurotransmitters in your brain which are norepinephrine and serotonin, and on a lesser level, dopamine. By blocking the re-uptake of these appetite-suppressing neurotransmitters, their levels stay higher in your brain. Higher neurotransmitter levels means that their signal lasts longer. The longer the signal lasts, the longer your sensation of fullness (and the lack of desire to eat) lasts.

Sibutramine may also work by decreasing cravings for carbohydrates. Carbohydrates boost levels of serotonin in the brain. Since sibutramine also boosts levels of serotonin in the brain, it may substitute for carbohydrates and thus curb cravings for carbohydrates. Finally, sibutramine also boosts adrenaline levels. Higher adrenaline levels may increase metabolism and diminish overall appetite. Sibutramine slows the usual decline in metabolism (normally occurring with weight loss) by about 100 calories per day.

Sibutramine is FDA-approved in doses of five to 15 mg/day in conjunction with a reduced-calorie diet. Studies of overweight patients taking sibutramine for at least eight weeks show greater weight loss over placebo, and after four to six months, average weight loss on sibutramine ranges from 7.5 to 13 pounds.[48] Year-long clinical trials show that sibutramine is also effective in long-term weight control, with individuals losing 10 pounds more (on average) than those receiving placebo. Based on these results, patients on sibutramine are 20 to 30 percent more likely to lose at least five percent of their body weight than those receiving placebo.

You may remember the market recall of fenfluramine (the fen half of the popular fen-phen drug combination) and Redux (dexfenfluramine) because of their link to potentially fatal heart valve abnormalities and primary pulmonary hypertension. You may be wondering how sibutramine is different. Although sibutramine and fenfluramine are similar in that they both affect serotonin in the brain, fenfluramine also boosts the levels of serotonin in the systemic blood stream. That is what is believed to have caused the heart valve damage seen in some patients. Sibutramine increases serotonin locally in the brain, but does not have a systemic effect (so should not be linked with heart valve damage). In other words, it bypasses the heart and acts directly on the appetite control center in the brain.

Though sibutramine may be safer than other anti-obesity drugs, it still warrants caution. The most concerning side effects include increased blood pressure and heart rate, and abnormal heart rhythms. Most of these side effects occur when large doses (more than 15 mg) are taken, and diminish when the dose is lowered. To be cautious, blood pressure and pulse measurements should be done before starting sibutramine and should be routinely monitored thereafter.

Other common side effects associated with sibutramine include dry mouth, headache, constipation, and insomnia. Sibutramine should not be taken if you are taking monoamine oxidase inhibitors (MAOIs), or other centrally acting weight loss agents. It should not be taken if you have an eating disorder (e.g., anorexia, bulimia), or if you are pregnant or nursing.

Orlistat (Xenical)

Orlistat (Xenical) is a gastrointestinal (GI) lipase inhibitor that is FDA approved for long-term weight control. It works in the body rather than the brain, where it blocks the breakdown of triglycerides (fat) into parts that can be absorbed. Orlistat causes weight loss by reducing the absorption of dietary fat by approximately 30 percent. An over-the-counter version of Orlistat, Alli is available as well at half of the dose. Since Medifast is a low-fat program, we do not recommend that you take Orlistat or Alli while on the plan.

Several long-term (one- to two-year long) studies show that orlistat is effective at causing a moderate amount of weight loss when compared to placebo. Individuals taking orlistat lost six to 10 percent of their total body weight compared with those on placebo who lost only about five percent.[49-56] The results of numerous studies showed that the average weight loss after one year of orlistat treatment was about six pounds more than those on placebo treatment. Orlistat also seems to be helpful in reducing the amount of weight that is regained after an initial weight-loss period.

In addition to its weight control benefits, long-term studies also show improvements in health outcomes. Reductions in total and LDL cholesterol, systolic and diastolic blood pressures, as well as fasting insulin and blood sugar levels among subjects with diabetes have been shown.

GI side effects are common with orlistat. They include flatulence with discharge, greasy stools, oily spotting, and fecal urgency, frequency, and even incontinence (particularly after high-fat meals). These effects tend to decrease with ongoing treatment. Adding natural fiber to your diet may reduce the frequency of these effects by absorbing water and adding bulk to stools. On the other hand, orlistat's effectiveness may be due (in part) to these GI side effects—if you know that eating a large, fatty meal or dessert will lead to unpleasant GI side effects when taking this medication, you may think twice before indulging.

Orlistat may also inhibit the absorption of some medications. For instance, decreased plasma levels of cyclosporine have been reported. In such patients, dose changes and monitoring of drug levels may be needed. It has also been shown to decrease the absorption of fat-soluble vitamins, so the daily use of multivitamins (particularly vitamin D) two hours before or after taking orlistat is recommended. People with chronic malabsorptive disorders or cholestasis should not take orlistat.

Combination (Sibutramine-Orlistat) therapy

A small study comparing sibutramine to orlistat found sibutramine alone, or in combination with orlistat, was more effective in reducing weight than orlistat alone.

FDA-approved for weight control (short term)

Phentermine

Short-term use of Phentermine (generally less than 12 weeks) is approved for weight loss. Phentermine works by stimulating norepinephrine and dopamine in the central nervous system (brain and nerves). By doing so, it increases metabolism and decreases appetite.

Studies suggest that appetite suppressing agents like phentermine are associated with moderate decreases in body weight when compared with placebo (four to 20 pounds). Few studies have looked into its longer-term effectiveness, that is, beyond six months.

While it was problematic when used in conjunction with fenfluramine, phentermine itself has not been associated with valvular heart disease. Typical side effects include insomnia, dry mouth, constipation, heart palpitations, high blood pressure, and euphoria (feelings of exaggerated well-being).

Phentermine may be habit forming, and physical and/or psychological dependence may occur. Withdrawal symptoms may occur if stopped suddenly after weeks of continuous use, so please talk to your doctor about discontinuing this medication gradually.

Individuals taking MAOIs, SSRIs, tricyclic antidepressants (TCAs), other weight-loss agents (including over-the-counter and herbal medications), or who drink alcohol, may not take phentermine. People with uncontrolled or poorly controlled blood pressure, symptoms of cardiovascular disease, anxiety, mania, glaucoma, hyperthyroidism, alcoholism, history of substance abuse or psychosis, or who are pregnant, breast-feeding, or younger than age 16 should not take phentermine.

Other (not FDA-approved for weight control)

Fluoxetine (Prozac)

Some studies suggest the antidepressant fluoxetine has short-term beneficial effects on body weight, but loses the weight-loss effect longer term. Fluoxetine may be of benefit in obese individuals who have other clinical disorders, such as binge eating or bulimia. However since fluoxetine appears to lose its body-weight reducing effect after six months, it does not appear to be a wise choice for long-term weight control in individuals who do not have other coexisting disorders.

Some side effects of fluoxetine include nausea, dry mouth, dizziness, anxiety, vivid dreams, ringing in the ears, sleeplessness, decreased libido, delayed or non-existent orgasm/ejaculation, heart palpitations, tremor, and restless legs.

Buproprion (Wellbutrin, Zyban)

Bupropion is FDA approved for the treatment of depression (Wellbutrin), as well as for smoking cessation (Zyban). While the exact mechanism of action is not fully known, bupropion works by blocking the re-uptake of norepinephrine and dopamine. Several studies have shown that this agent is associated with weight loss in obese individuals both with and without depression. Obese adults with symptoms of depression taking 300 mg of bupropion SR per day were shown to lose an average of about 10 pounds, compared to about four pounds in those on placebo at the end of six months. Adults without depression similarly lost weight on bupropion when combined with a low calorie diet using two meal replacements per day for six months. Individuals on bupropion SR 300 mg per day, 400 mg per day, or placebo, lost seven, 10, and five percent of their body weight, respectively.[57]

Some individuals who take bupropion have GI upset (e.g., nausea, vomiting, abdominal pain), CNS effects (e.g., trembling, blurred vision, agitation, headache, hallucinations, seizures), and cardiovascular effects (e.g., irregular heart beats). This drug may be most helpful in obese individuals who are depressed, who desire smoking cessation, or both.

Zonisamide (Zonegran)

Zonisamide is currently approved as an anti-seizure medication. It appears to work by blocking sodium and calcium channels. It also has effects on dopamine, serotonin, and carbonic anhydrase, which may suppress appetite. A short-term clinical trial (16-weeks) involving 60 patients (mostly women) showed a six percent weight loss in patients on zonisamide compared to a one percent weight loss in placebo-treated patients.[58] In 36 patients who completed 16 more weeks of the study, the mean total weight loss was about 18 pounds. Some CNS side effects like fatigue and dizziness have been reported in studies on this drug. In rare instances, kidney stones and hematologic events have also been noted. With the appropriate person (e.g., obese with epilepsy, obese with depression), zonisamide may play a role in helping reduce body weight.

Topiramate (Topamax)

Topiramate is currently approved as an add-on treatment for seizure disorders. Both animal and human studies have demonstrated weight loss with this agent. Studies of topiramate-treated patients show a total body weight percentage loss of eight percent.[59-61] GI and CNS side effects have been reported. This drug, like zonisamide, may have a role in select individuals (e.g., obese with epilepsy, obese with depression).

Weight-loss agents and Medifast

You can use weight-loss agents while on Medifast. A December 2005 study in the New England Journal of Medicine showed that individuals who lost the most weight after one year are those who combine diet and lifestyle modification with weight-loss medication (sibutramine).[62]

Let's see how Medifast plus a weight-loss agent may be more effective than either alone. Medifast, in and of itself, is designed to be satiating (cause fullness) due to its higher protein and fiber content. So the combination of Medifast plus appetite suppression therapy may maximally decrease appetite so that fewer calories are consumed. This may work best in individuals who are struggling with physical feelings of hunger (e.g., hunger pangs) on Medifast alone.

In addition to helping reduce the amount of calorie intake, the other added benefit of appetite suppression therapy is that many of these agents also increase the number of calories burned (calories out), or at least prevent the reduction in metabolism that normally occurs with weight loss. Recall that sibutramine has been shown to decrease the reduction in energy expenditure by 100 calories per day.

Each calorie that comes in and each calorie that goes out, counts when you are trying to lose weight. Remember the energy balance equation:

Calories In < Calories Out = Weight Loss

By combining Medifast with an appetite suppressant, there will be two treatments working to reduce your caloric intake (Medifast and the appetite suppressant agent), and one working to increase the number of calories out (the appetite suppressant agent). Reducing the number of calories in and increasing the number of calories out may yield maximal weight loss results by working at both ends of the energy balance equation.

Medifast may be used with any of the appetite suppressant medications aforementioned; however the Medifast Program alone naturally suppresses appetite and eliminates hunger without requiring other therapies (for most people). Please consult your primary healthcare provider for more information on the use of weight-loss medications and Medifast.

Weight-loss surgery

When dietary and medicinal approaches to weight loss fail, people start looking to more extreme measures of weight control. Bariatric (gastrointestinal) surgery is a more extreme weight control tactic, reserved for patients with severe obesity who have failed diet/medical therapy (and are suffering from its complications). Bariatric surgery is generally regarded as the most effective obesity treatment available. However, despite its effectiveness, the stakes are also very high when it comes to surgical risks and complications, which may even lead to death. Because surgery is high risk, it is generally only recommended for highly motivated patients with acceptable operative risks. It is not recommended for patients with unacceptable operative risks, or for those who are not motivated to make the strict post-operative diet and lifestyle changes necessary for weight loss. To be considered a candidate for bariatric surgery you must have a BMI (kg/m2) of at least:

35 plus serious obesity-related health conditions
(e.g., high blood pressure, high cholesterol, type 2 diabetes)

OR

40 without obesity-related health conditions

Types of surgery

There are three types of bariatric surgery performed for weight loss: restrictive, malabsorptive, and restrictive-malabsorptive. Since Roux-en-Y gastric bypass (RGB) surgery is the most commonly performed bariatric procedure in the U.S., and considered to be the gold standard, it is the surgical technique that we will discuss further.

RGB is a restrictive-malabsorptive type of surgery. The stomach is reduced to the size of a small stomach pouch in order to restrict food intake. Then, a Y-shaped section of the small intestine is attached to the pouch to allow food to bypass parts of the digestive tract so that the amount of calories and nutrients the body can absorb is restricted. Because the new stomach pouch is very small and most of the stomach and small intestine have been bypassed, there are normal consequences that occur as a result. Some consequences to expect after gastric bypass surgery include:

- Permanent food intake restriction
- Decreased absorption of vitamins and minerals (e.g., iron, vitamin B12, calcium)
- Dumping syndrome
  May occur if foods and liquids (mostly high-sugar or high-carbohydrate types) enter your small intestine rapidly leading to nausea, vomiting, diarrhea, dizziness, rapid heart beats, and sweating.
- Lactose intolerance
  Lactose is the natural sugar found in milk and milk products that is digested in the small bowel by the enzyme lactase. Lactose intolerance occurs in individuals who do not have enough lactase to digest milk. So when milk-based products are consumed, crampy abdominal pain, gas, and diarrhea may result. Lactose intolerance is acquired after gastric bypass in about 10 percent of patients.
- Temporary body adjustments to rapid weight loss (e.g., thinning of the hair, dry skin, fatigue, joint aches, mood changes)
- Life-long medical follow-up
- Psychological adjustments to the new body weight and size

Benefits

Weight loss is immediate and substantial with gastric bypass surgery. Approximately 75 percent of patients may lose 75 to 80 percent of their excess body weight, and the weight loss may be maintained for several years. Health problems (e.g., type 2 diabetes mellitus, high blood pressure, osteoarthritis) related to the obesity are often improved as well. About 70 to 80 percent of patients with high blood pressure, and over 90 percent of patients with diabetes are able to discontinue their medications. Individuals may have significant reductions in heart disease, lung disease, and certain cancers. Furthermore, sleep apnea, joint pain, heartburn, fatigue, shortness of breath, quality of life, and self-esteem may all be improved.

Perhaps most significantly, researchers have shown that morbidly obese individuals who underwent gastric bypass surgery had an 89 percent lower chance of dying in five years compared with morbidly obese persons who did not.

Risks

Despite these significant benefits, remember that gastric bypass is a major surgery with dangers of its own. Some risks associated with gastric bypass surgery include infection, suture/staple line leaks, incisional hernias, heart arrhythmias, and pneumonia. The death rate from gastric bypass surgery is approximately one out of 350 people when performed by an experienced surgeon. The death rate may be higher, however, if the surgeon is less experienced in performing gastric bypass procedures.

Nutritional deficiencies may occur as a result of gastric bypass surgery because the operation bypasses much of the small intestine where many nutrients are absorbed. Iron, vitamin B12, and folate deficiencies may occur, leading to anemia. Also, calcium absorption may be decreased, leading to osteoporosis or osteomalacia (softening of the bones). A thiamin (B1) deficiency may also be a concern if B1 dietary sources (e.g., legumes, peas, nuts, beef) cannot be consumed after surgery. To prevent deficiencies, it is essential that patients take nutritional supplements.

Gastric bypass

Diet and lifestyle changes after gastric bypass surgery

What you eat, how you eat, and how much you eat change after gastric bypass surgery because the operation has altered the anatomy of your digestive system. The volume that the new stomach pouch can hold is reduced from about one quart to approximately one ounce (or two tablespoons). Over time, the stomach pouch will stretch until it can hold about four to eight ounces (½ to 1 cup) at a time. Since the size of the opening created between the stomach and small intestine is smaller now, it slows the rate at which food is emptied from the stomach into the small intestine. With your stomach pouch reduced to the size of a walnut, you'll need to follow a gastric-bypass diet that will help you maintain good nutrition while losing weight. A doctor or dietitian will help you create a meal plan consisting of the right type, amount, and consistency/textures of foods.

In addition to taking vitamin and mineral supplementation (multivitamin, iron, calcium, vitamin B12), there are other general dietary guidelines to follow after gastric bypass surgery. Meals and snacks should be:

- Small and frequent
- High in protein
- Low in calories, fat, and sugar
- Low-lactose (for some)
- Fortified with vitamin & minerals

You can see that Medifast meets each and every nutritional requirement of the gastric bypass surgery diet.

The first three months after surgery

After surgery, you will not be allowed to eat for one to two days. In most cases, liquids will be the first food introduced to your new stomach. A liquid diet is generally followed for about two to three days. During this time, foods and fluids that are mostly water and liquid at room temperature may be consumed. They include things like broth, juice, and cereal.

After this initial phase, you will begin what is referred to as a diet progression. The purpose of a diet progression is to allow your new stomach time to adapt to processing foods. Because your stomach is still healing, you will progress to a pureed diet for about three to four weeks. Pureed foods have the consistency of a smooth paste or thick liquid. After that, you can progress to a soft foods diet for about eight weeks. Soft foods include items that can be easily chewed like cooked vegetables, diced or ground meats, and softened or canned fruits. The soft foods diet should be followed for about eight weeks before progressing to a regular foods diet.

During the diet progression, it is recommended that you eat six small meals per day and sip water frequently. Then you may progress to eating four meals per day, and finally decrease to eating three meals and three snacks per day. Protein-rich foods are recommended during the diet progression. Medifast Meals and snacks (e.g., shakes, oatmeals, puddings) may be particularly helpful during this phase by providing the right texture (liquid, soft) as well as the necessary protein, vitamins, and minerals that your healing body needs. You should discuss with your doctor or dietitian about how you may incorporate Medifast into your diet progression.

Lifelong changes (after three months)

After three months, it is generally recommended that you eat three small meals and three small, healthy snacks a day. Your meal composition should be low in calories, fat, and sugar, but high in protein. Since Medifast is portion-controlled, and consists of the same meal composition that is often recommended after gastric bypass surgery, it may help aid in your continued weight loss, as well as make the new diet easier to stick to.

Medifast provides small, frequent, portion-controlled Meals

Though your stomach stretches over time to hold more food, you will likely not be able to eat more than one to one-and-a-half cups of food during each meal. Eating too much food adds extra calories and can cause pain, nausea, vomiting and abdominal cramps. Since the stomach can only handle very small amounts of food, it is important to eat the right portions of nutritionally sound foods frequently after surgery to ensure meeting nutritional requirements.

Medifast Meals are high in protein

Getting enough protein is important after gastric bypass surgery in both the short- and long-run. Since the body needs to build new tissue and ensure wounds heal properly after surgery, it is important to get enough protein right after surgery. Medifast Meals are an excellent source of protein and are also low in calories, sugar, and carbohydrates.

Medifast Meals are low-glycemic (low in carbs and sugar)

There are three reasons to avoid sugar after gastric bypass surgery. First, these foods tend to be high in calories and fat. Even in moderate amounts, they could make weight loss difficult. Second, eating sweet or sugary foods promotes dumping syndrome. Experiencing the unpleasant symptoms of dumping syndrome may limit the desire to eat sweet foods. With Medifast you are likely to avoid these unpleasant symptoms. Third, most sweet and sugary foods don't provide many vitamins or minerals for the calories they contain.

Medifast Meals are low in fat

In addition to being high in calories, fat may be difficult to digest after gastric bypass surgery. Too much fat delays the emptying of the stomach and may cause gastroesophageal reflux, a back-up of stomach acid and food into the esophagus that causes heartburn. Fat may also lead to diarrhea, nausea, or stomach discomfort.

Many Medifast Meals are lactose-free

For the 10 percent of individuals who have a lactose intolerance after gastric bypass surgery, look for Medifast products that are low-lactose or lactose-free. That way, unpleasant side effects, (e.g., bloating, flatulence, cramping) due to lactose, can be avoided.

Medifast Meals are fortified with vitamins & minerals

Vitamins and minerals are an important part of the gastric bypass diet. Since the diet allows only small amounts of a limited variety of foods, it may be difficult to get enough vitamins and minerals from food alone. Deficiencies can develop in a matter of months, with iron, folate, vitamin B-12, and/or calcium, the nutrients most often affected. For this reason, multivitamin/mineral supplementation is recommended. Another way you can ensure an adequate intake of nutrients (in addition to taking vitamin/mineral supplements) is through Medifast, since Medifast Meals are vitamin and mineral fortified.

Weight maintenance

Having bariatric surgery is not a guarantee of long-term weight control success. In order to maintain weight loss, you can not return to your old eating habits. If you do, you may regain all of the weight back that you previously had lost. People who regain weight after gastric bypass surgery usually are consuming too many high-calorie foods and beverages. Medifast can be used during the Maintenance phase to prevent this from happening, as you will need to watch portions, calories, fats, and sugars for life. With Medifast, your new dietary and lifestyle requirements after gastric bypass surgery may be more easily achieved and maintained.

This chapter has informed you about medications and surgery for weight control. You have learned that drugs and surgery can cause weight loss (although risks are high), and that Medifast's structured meal program is also a potent weight control intervention, with low risks. Some people really do need the added benefit of medications and/or surgery. Many do not. Despite which group of people you fall into, Medifast can help.

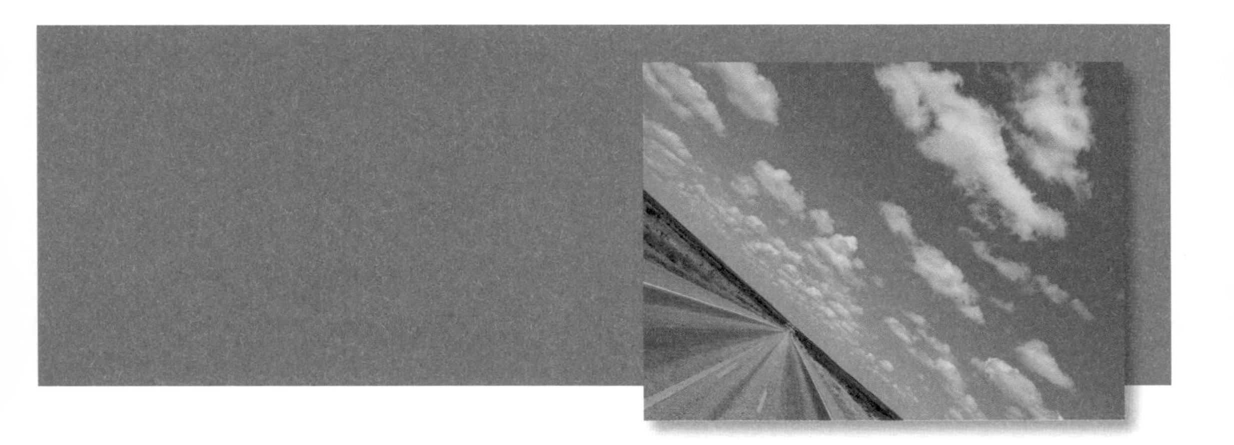

14 On your way

This book has provided you with a great deal of information. You learned about the causes of the obesity epidemic in the first part of the book. You learned what to watch for in the fat-promoting environment—and who the friends and foes of your weight-control efforts are. You learned that obesity is not only a cosmetic problem, but a major health problem as well. The major health consequences associated with obesity may not affect us while we're young, but they certainly begin affecting us as we age. You also learned that there are important differences between men and women when it comes to health and weight control, and that Medifast's nutritionally enhanced meals were designed to meet the needs of both.

Medifast takes advantage of scientific research that demonstrates how we can most effectively change eating patterns, and gain control of our weight with a minimal amount of discomfort. You learned that eating small, frequent meals is better than eating large meals, and (contrary to popular knowledge) protein is more filling than fat. You also learned some strategic weight control tools like how to mindfully eat your meals.

You learned that in addition to exercise, Medifast Meals can help you stay healthy for life and maintain control over your weight. Other big take home points are that the use of soy protein provides significant health benefits that other proteins and diets do not. And that Medifast may be used as the sole weight control tactic, or in combination with more extreme weight control measures (like weight-loss medications and gastric bypass surgery).

We visited a number of people who successfully lost weight with Medifast. They come from all walks of life, with a variety of motivations and goals. They lost a lot of weight, improved their health, and improved their outlook on life. They provide inspiration and guidance, even though they may not be typical or reflect your exact situation and needs.

The Medifast Program was designed by a physician with you in mind, and Medifast is ready to provide you with support and guidance on your program. Medifast has been *the doctor's secret* to successful weight loss for over 25 years. Now the secret is out—and while the path is not always easy, we hope that lessons learned from this book will be helpful to you along your Medifast journey.

Good Luck!

Ron Taylor

lost 109 pounds with Medifast

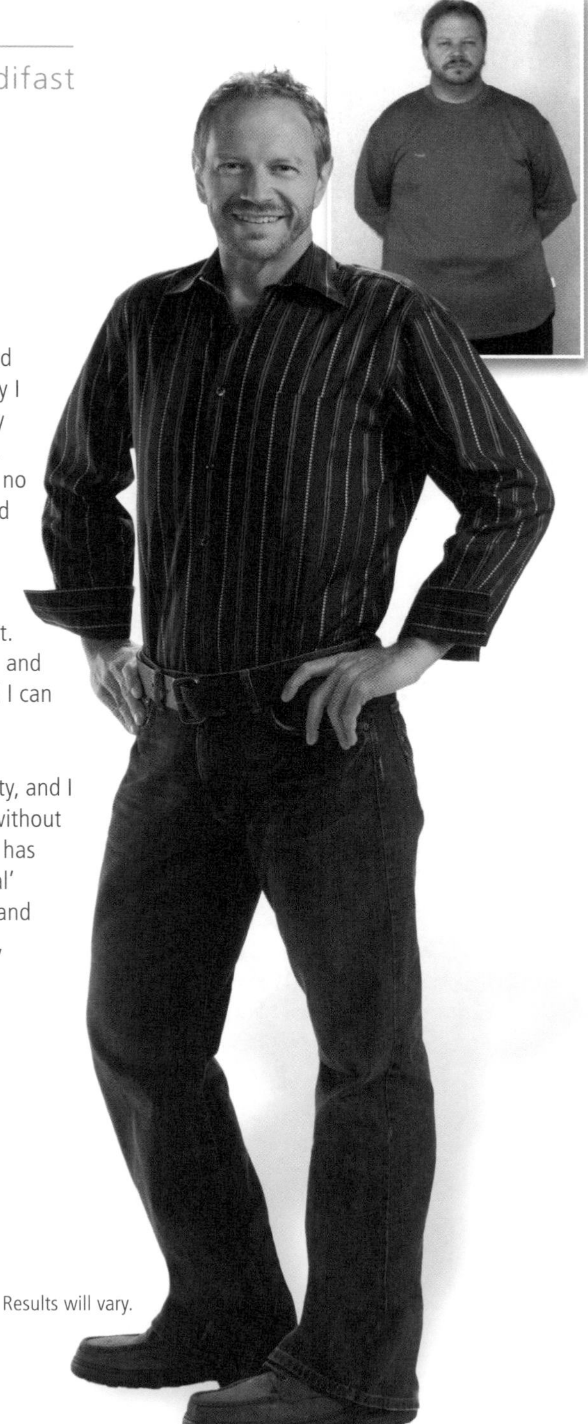

"I used to be 302 pounds, with slight hypertension and no self-confidence. I had limited mobility and just knowing the way I looked (FAT) made me feel depressed. My weight problem affected everything I did, from work to my social life. I had little to no success with fad dieting. I ALWAYS gained back the weight I lost—plus some.

"I heard about Medifast Weight Control Centers on the radio, and decided to try it. Within the first few days I already looked and felt better. Now, I weigh 193 pounds and I can easily fit into smaller sizes and spaces!

"I have so much more energy and mobility, and I can now do everyday physical activities without getting out of breath. My blood pressure has normalized and I finally feel like a 'normal' person. My weight loss occurred quickly and dramatically, and all of my friends, family, and co-workers immediately noticed a difference. They have all been very supportive and have shared in my joy."

Results will vary.

This success story lost weight using a Medifast Weight Control Centers Program.

Nnedi Uzihowe

lost 170 pounds with Medifast

"After the birth of my daughter, I realized that I gained a lot of weight. I was placed on bed rest and gained 70 pounds during the pregnancy. Three months post-delivery I decided to do something about it. I had seen an ad about Medifast and I decided to give it a try; boy am I glad I did.

"Within 5 months I had lost a total of 92 pounds. My energy had gone up, I was not hungry, and, most of all, Medifast tastes great. My favorite flavor is Strawberry Creme. I like to mix it and leave it in the freezer for 30 minutes. Then I eat it with a spoon.

"To think that I had even considered gastric bypass is scary. I am so glad I never went that route. Medifast is so easy to follow, just shake and drink; no measuring and no counting. I would recommend this to anyone who has been battling with his or her weight."

Results will vary.

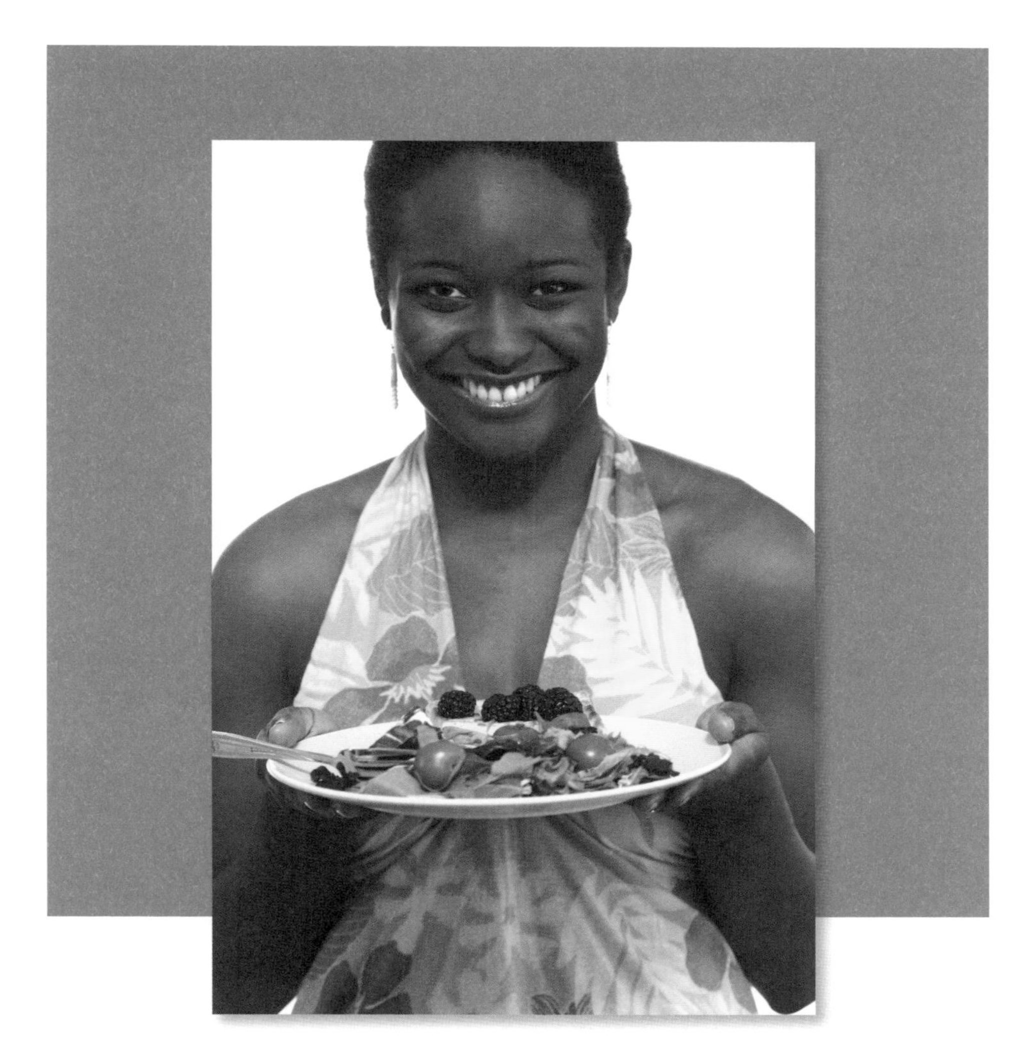

15 Recipes and Meal Plans

The Medifast program is easy, convenient and fits in with your busy lifestyle. Included in this section is a sampling of great recipes for your Lean & Green Meal as well as calorie-free ways to spice up your Medifast Meals. We have also included several sample meal plans. There are lots of ways to have fun with the Medifast program, so experiment and try all of the different foods and recipes available.

Lean & Green Recipes

Grilled Cajun Turkey Tenderloins

Serves: 4 *Preparation Time:* 10 minutes *Cook Time:* 20 minutes

28 oz (raw) boneless turkey breast tenderloins
6 cups romaine lettuce
6 cups raw spinach
¼ cup low-fat, low-carbohydrate sun-dried tomato salad dressing

Seasoning Rub:
4 tsp extra virgin olive oil
1-½ tsp paprika
½ tsp onion powder
½ tsp cayenne powder
¼ tsp garlic powder

Instructions:

Combine all ingredients for the seasoning rub in a bowl. Rub turkey tenderloins evenly with spice mixture.

Place turkey on grill and cook for 5-10 minutes per side or until turkey is thoroughly cooked (meat thermometer should read 170°F).

Toss lettuce, spinach, and dressing together. Serve with turkey tenderloins.

Per Serving: *(Serving is approximately 6 oz cooked turkey tenderloins and 3 cups salad greens.)*

310 calories	10 g fat	80 mg cholesterol
330 mg sodium	7 g total carbs	3 g fiber
51 g protein		

(Count as 2 optional condiments per serving.)

Balsamic-Glazed Chicken Breast

Serves: 4 *Preparation Time:* 15 minutes (plus at least 3 hours marinating)
Cook Time: 45-60 minutes

4 8-oz (raw) boneless, skinless chicken breasts or strips
6 cups broccoli
⅛ cup water
2 Tbsp balsamic vinegar
1 Tbsp extra virgin olive oil

Seasoning Rub:
4 Tbsp fresh rosemary leaves, chopped
2 Tbsp water
2 cloves garlic, minced
1 tsp black pepper
1 tsp extra virgin olive oil

Instructions:

To make seasoning rub: Combine the garlic, rosemary, black pepper, water, and olive oil. Rinse chicken and pat dry. Rub the chicken with mixture, then cover and refrigerate for 3 hours or overnight.

Preheat oven to 350°F. While oven warms, combine ⅛ cup water, 2 Tbsp balsamic vinegar, and 1 Tbsp extra virgin olive oil. Pour half this mixture in the bottom of a small roasting pan. Place chicken breasts in pan and pour remaining balsamic vinegar mixture over chicken. Roast in the oven for 45 minutes or until cooked thoroughly. Steam broccoli and serve on the side.

Per Serving: *(Serving is approximately 6 oz cooked chicken breast and 1-½ cups broccoli.)*

330 calories	10 g fat	125 mg cholesterol
160 mg sodium	10 g total carbs	4 g fiber
49 g protein		

(Count as 3 optional condiments per serving.)

Taco Salad

Serves: 1 *Preparation Time:* 5 minutes *Cook Time:* 20 minutes

7-½ oz (raw) ground beef or turkey (95-97% fat-free)
1 cup romaine lettuce
1 cup iceberg lettuce
½ cup tomatoes, diced
2 Tbsp salsa
1 Tbsp water
¾ tsp taco seasoning (low-sodium versions preferred)

Instructions:

Brown ground turkey or beef in a pan. Drain grease; add 1 Tbsp water and taco seasoning to meat in pan. Simmer on low heat for 5 minutes.

Prepare plate with the 2 cups of mixed lettuce (romaine and iceberg) and diced tomatoes. Top salad mix with ground turkey or beef and salsa.

Per Serving:

330 calories	11 g fat	130 mg cholesterol
480 mg sodium	11 g total carbs	3 g fiber
44 g protein		

(Count as 3 optional condiments per serving.)

Green Bean Almondine

Serves: 4

1-½ lbs raw green beans, trimmed
4 Tbsp almonds, slivered
2 Tbsp butter
Salt and pepper (to taste)

Instructions:

Saute almonds in butter until lightly browned; be careful not to burn. Steam green beans. Toss with almonds and season with salt and pepper before serving.

Per Serving:

148 calories	10 g fat	15 mg cholesterol
5 g protein	15 g total carbs	

(Count as 3 Greens (vegetables) and 2 Healthy Fats per serving.)

Grilled Halibut with Lemon Vinaigrette

Serves: 1 ***Preparation Time:*** 20 minutes ***Cook Time:*** 15 minutes

7 oz (raw) halibut filet
½ cup fresh or frozen green beans
½ cup fresh or frozen broccoli
½ cup fresh or frozen cauliflower
Salt and pepper (to taste)

Vinaigrette:
2 tsp lemon juice
2 tsp olive oil
1 tsp chopped capers
¾ tsp finely chopped shallots or green onions
Salt and pepper (to taste)

Instructions:

Combine all ingredients for the vinaigrette in a small bowl and whisk.

Coat a non-stick grill pan with cooking spray and heat over medium heat. If desired, sprinkle fish with salt and pepper on both sides and lay on grill pan. Cook 3-5 minutes on each side or until thoroughly cooked.

Steam green beans, broccoli, and cauliflower.

Spoon vinaigrette onto fish. Serve with steamed vegetables.

Per Serving: *(Serving is approximately 6 oz cooked halibut and 1-½ cups steamed vegetables.)*

340 calories	14 g fat	65 mg cholesterol
220 mg sodium	10 g total carbs	5 g fiber
44 g protein		

(Count as 3 optional condiments per serving.)

Herb-roasted Turkey Breast

Serves: 2   ***Preparation Time:*** 30 minutes   ***Cook Time:*** 45-60 minutes

1 lb (16 oz) boneless turkey breast, raw
2 cups celery, chopped
1 cup mushrooms, sliced
2 Tbsp onion, diced
1 tsp poultry seasoning
½ tsp ground black pepper
½ cup low-sodium chicken broth
½ tsp onion powder
½ tsp garlic powder
2 tsp canola oil, butter, or trans fat-free margarine

Instructions:

Preheat oven to 350° F. Place turkey breasts in medium roasting pan. Sprinkle equal amounts of poultry seasoning, black pepper, onion and garlic powder on turkey breasts.

Place celery, onions, and sliced mushrooms around turkey breasts. Pour chicken broth and oil (or butter/trans fat-free margarine) into roasting pan. Roast for 45-60 minutes or until internal temperature of turkey breasts reaches 170° F.

If cooking turkey breasts with skin on, remove skin prioir to eating.

Per Serving: *(Serving is approximately 6 oz cooked turkey and 1-½ cups mixed vegetables.)*

323 calories	7 g fat	148 mg cholesterol
56 g protein	7 g total carbs	

(Count as 1 full Lean & Green Meal (6 oz "leaner" Lean choice, 3 Green, and 1 Healthy Fat) and 2 optional condiments per serving.)

Medifast Meal Recipes

Chinese Soup

Serves: 1

1 Medifast Chicken Noodle Soup
1 cup (8 oz) water
2 tsp regular or low-sodium soy sauce
1 tsp hot/Chinese mustard

Instructions:

Empty contents of Medifast Chicken Noodle Soup into a deep microwave-safe bowl and add 1 cup water; stir. Mix soy sauce and mustard into soup. Microwave for 2-½ minutes. Let stand for 1 minute and stir. Microwave again for 1 minute (watching it doesn't boil over). Take out of microwave, cover, and let stand 3-5 minutes (the steam will cook it the rest of the way). Do NOT prepare in a shaker jar.

(Count as 1 Medifast Meal and 3 optional condiments per serving.)

Shake Cookies

Serves: 1 (makes approximately 3-5 cookies)

1 Medifast French Vanilla 55 or 70 Shake
⅛ tsp baking powder
2 packets (or 2 tsp) Splenda® Sweetener
½ tsp vanilla extract
½ tsp ground cinnamon
¼ cup water

Instructions:

Preheat oven to 350° F. Combine all ingredients in a bowl. Spray a foil-lined, oven-safe pan with non-stick cooking spray. Drop mixture by teaspoon onto the pan and bake for about 15 minutes.

Per Serving: *(based on the Medifast French Vanilla 55 Shake)*

100 calories	0.5 g fat	0 mg cholesterol
11 g protein	16 g total carbs	

(Count as 1 Medifast Meal and 3 optional condiments per serving.)

Hot Cocoa Viennese

Serves: 1

1 Medifast Hot Cocoa
½ tsp ground cinnamon
6 oz hot water
¼ tsp vanilla extract

Instructions:

Combine Hot Cocoa and cinnamon in a mug or microwave-safe cup. Add hot water and vanilla extract; stir until dissolved. Allow drink to cool for a few minutes to blend flavors, then stir again and enjoy.

Per Serving:

115 calories	1 g fat	10 mg cholesterol
14 g protein	15 g total carbs	

(Count as 1 Medifast Meal and 1 optional condiment per serving.)

Cinnabon Shake

Serves: 1

1 Medifast French Vanilla 55 or 70 Shake
1 tsp ButterBuds®
½ tsp ground cinnamon
½ cup cold water
¼ cup ice

Instructions:

Pour ingredients into blender and mix until smooth.

Per Serving: *(based on the Medifast French Vanilla 55 Shake)*

97 calories	0.5 g fat	0 mg cholesterol
11 g protein	16 g total carbs	

(Count as 1 Medifast Meal and 3 optional condiments per serving.)

5 & 1 Meal Plans

The following meal plans are appropriate for anyone following the Medifast 5 & 1 Plan. All meal plans should include at least **eight** 8-ounce glasses of water (64 ounces total) each day.

Day 1

BREAKFAST *1ST Medifast Meal*	Medifast Scrambled Eggs with a sprinkle of dill*
MID-MORNING *2ND Medifast Meal*	Medifast Cappuccino
LUNCH *3RD Medifast Meal*	Medifast Chicken Noodle Soup
MID-AFTERNOON *4TH Medifast Meal*	Medifast Chocolate Mint Crunch Bar
DINNER *Lean & Green Meal*	• 6 oz chicken breast, grilled on a kabob with 1 cup mix of green, yellow, and red peppers and ½ cup mix of yellow squash, cherry tomatoes, and zucchini • Brush kabobs with 1 tsp olive oil** and ½ tsp barbeque sauce*
EVENING *5TH Medifast Meal*	Medifast Chocolate Pudding

*optional condiment **healthy fat serving

5 & 1 Meal Plans

All meal plans should include at least **eight** 8-ounce glasses of water (64 ounces total) each day.

Day 2

BREAKFAST *1ST Medifast Meal*	Medifast Strawberry Crème Shake blended with ice for a "smoothie"
MID-MORNING *2ND Medifast Meal*	Medifast Apple Cinnamon Oatmeal with a dash of extra cinnamon* on top
LUNCH *Lean & Green Meal*	• 5 oz flame-grilled sirloin steak smothered with ½ cup cooked mushrooms and 1 tsp A1 Steak Sauce®* drizzled on top • ½ cup cabbage sprinkled with cayenne pepper* • ½ cup asparagus with 5 sprays of non-caloric imitation butter*
MID-AFTERNOON *3RD Medifast Meal*	Medifast Chicken & Wild Rice Soup
DINNER *4TH Medifast Meal*	Medifast Chai Latté
EVENING *5TH Medifast Meal*	Medifast Cranberry Mango Fruit Drink

*optional condiment

5 & 1 Meal Plans

All meal plans should include at least **eight** 8-ounce glasses of water (64 ounces total) each day.

Day 3	
BREAKFAST *Lean & Green Meal*	• 2 cups egg substitute, cooked in 2 tsp canola oil** • Sautée 1 cup mix of green and red peppers and ½ cup cooked spinach • Top with 1 Tbsp salsa* for a fiesta omelet
MID-MORNING *1ST Medifast Meal*	Medifast Swiss Mocha Shake
LUNCH *2ND Medifast Meal*	Medifast Fruit & Nut Crunch Bar
MID-AFTERNOON *3RD Medifast Meal*	Medifast Homestyle Chili with a dash of Tabasco® sauce* and sprinkle of chili powder*
DINNER *4TH Medifast Meal*	Medifast Peach Iced Tea
EVENING *5TH Medifast Meal*	Medifast Banana Pudding

*optional condiment **healthy fat serving

5 & 1 Meal Plans

All meal plans should include at least **eight** 8-ounce glasses of water (64 ounces total) each day.

Day 4

BREAKFAST *1ST Medifast Meal*	Medifast Hot Cocoa blended with coffee and ice for a "frappe"
MID-MORNING *2ND Medifast Meal*	Medifast Maple & Brown Sugar Oatmeal
LUNCH *3RD Medifast Meal and Lean & Green Meal (1st half)* *(½ with the lunch meal and ½ with the dinner meal)*	Medifast Vanilla Pudding • 3 oz pan-seared fresh tilapia • 1 cup salad greens with ½ cup mix of diced tomatoes, radishes, and cucumbers • Drizzle with 1 tsp olive oil** and a squeeze of lemon*
MID-AFTERNOON *4TH Medifast Meal*	Medifast Raspberry Iced Tea
DINNER *Lean & Green Meal (2nd half)*	• 4 oz freshly steamed lobster tail dipped in 1 tsp trans fat-free margarine** • ½ cup mix of raw broccoli and cauliflower
EVENING *5TH Medifast Meal*	Medifast Orange Crème Shake (freeze and eat with a spoon for a special treat)

*optional condiment **healthy fat serving

5 & 1 Meal Plans

All meal plans should include at least **eight** 8-ounce glasses of water (64 ounces total) each day.

Day 5

BREAKFAST *1ST Medifast Meal*	Medifast Blueberry Oatmeal and 1 cup of coffee with 1 Tbsp skim milk*
MID-MORNING *2ND Medifast Meal*	Medifast Tropical Punch Fruit Drink • 3 celery stalks *(healthy snack)*
LUNCH *3RD Medifast Meal*	Medifast Beef Vegetable Stew
MID-AFTERNOON *4TH Medifast Meal*	Medifast Caramel Crunch Bar
DINNER *Lean & Green Meal* *(with Lean portion divided into two choices, totaling 7 oz of lean seafood choices)*	• 3 oz cold shrimp with 1 tsp cocktail sauce* • 4 oz baked orange roughy • 1 cup steamed green beans • ½ cup spaghetti squash cooked in 2 tsp of trans fat-free margarine** with cinnamon* and/or artificial sweetener* to taste
EVENING *5TH Medifast Meal*	Medifast Dutch Chocolate Shake

*optional condiment **healthy fat serving

5 & 1 Meal Plans

All meal plans should include at least **eight** 8-ounce glasses of water (64 ounces total) each day.

Meal Plan for Women

BREAKFAST *1ST Medifast Meal*	Medifast Ready-to-Drink Dutch Chocolate Shake
MID-MORNING *2ND Medifast Meal*	Medifast Scrambled Eggs with a dash of parsley*
LUNCH *Lean & Green Meal (1st half)* *(with Green divided between lunch and dinner meals, total of 3 servings)*	• 6 oz roasted turkey • 1 cup steamed mustard greens topped with 1 tsp olive oil** and salt* and pepper* to taste
MID-AFTERNOON *3RD Medifast Meal*	Medifast Strawberry Crème 55 Shake blended with ice and water
DINNER *4TH Medifast Meal and Lean & Green Meal (2nd half)*	Medifast Cream of Broccoli Soup with ½ cup steamed broccoli for added texture
EVENING *5TH Medifast Meal*	Medifast Plus for Women's Health Vanilla Shake

*optional condiment **healthy fat serving

5 & 1 Meal Plans

All meal plans should include at least **eight** 8-ounce glasses of water (64 ounces total) each day.

Meal Plan for Men

BREAKFAST *1ST Medifast Meal*	Medifast Blueberry Oatmeal
MID-MORNING *2ND Medifast Meal*	Medifast Banana Crème 70 Shake
LUNCH *3RD Medifast Meal*	Medifast Cream of Chicken Soup
MID-AFTERNOON *4TH Medifast Meal*	Medifast Chocolate Crunch Bar
DINNER *Lean & Green Meal*	• 5 oz slow cooked roast beef with 1 clove garlic*, minced, for taste • 1-½ cups mix of cooked tomatoes, green peppers, mushrooms, turnips, and/or zucchini
EVENING *5TH Medifast Meal*	Medifast French Vanilla 70 Shake

*optional condiment **healthy fat serving

5 & 1 Meal Plans

All meal plans should include at least **eight** 8-ounce glasses of water (64 ounces total) each day.

Meatless Meal Option

BREAKFAST *1ST Medifast Meal*	Medifast Swiss Mocha Shake mixed with ice and coffee for a "frappe"
MID-MORNING *2ND Medifast Meal*	Medifast Blueberry Oatmeal with 5 drops of pure vanilla extract*
LUNCH *3RD Medifast Meal*	Medifast Cream of Tomato Soup
MID-AFTERNOON *4TH Medifast Meal*	Medifast Dutch Chocolate 70 Shake
DINNER *Lean & Green Meal*	• 15 oz extra-firm tofu • 1 cup salad greens with 1 cup mix of diced tomatoes, green peppers, and raw broccoli • Drizzle with 2 tsp olive oil** and 1 tsp balsamic vinegar*
EVENING *5TH Medifast Meal*	Medifast Oatmeal Raisin Crunch Bar

*optional condiment **healthy fat serving

5 & 1 Meal Plans

All meal plans should include at least **eight** 8-ounce glasses of water (64 ounces total) each day.

Meal Plan for the Daily Exerciser	
BREAKFAST *1ST Medifast Meal*	Medifast Scrambled Eggs with a splash of Tabasco® sauce*
MID-MORNING *2ND Medifast Meal*	Medifast Maple & Brown Sugar Oatmeal • 1 cup unsweetened brewed tea with a splash of lemon*
LUNCH *Lean & Green Meal (first half)* *(divided into two portions: ½ as the lunch meal and ½ with the dinner meal)*	• 3 oz baked chicken breast brushed with 1 tsp teriyaki sauce* • 1 cup steamed green beans
MID-AFTERNOON *3RD Medifast Meal*	Medifast Lemon Meringue Crunch Bar
DINNER *4TH Medifast Meal and Lean & Green Meal*	Medifast Chocolate Pudding • 3 oz grilled swordfish • ½ cup steamed broccoli topped with 1 tsp trans fat-free margarine**
EVENING *5TH Medifast Meal*	Medifast Orange Creme 70 Shake stirred into diet lemon-lime or cream soda *(do not use shaker jar)*

*optional condiment **healthy fat serving

4 & 2 & 1 Meal Plan

If you have diabetes, your physician may recommend a meal plan that is higher in calories that the typical meal plan below. The sample higher-calorie meal plan option (on the next page) may be more appropriate for you. Talk to your doctor about which meal plan is right for you. All meal plans should include at least **eight** 8-ounce glasses of water (64 ounces total) each day.

Meal Plan for People with Diabetes
(taken from the Medifast for Diabetes Guide)

BREAKFAST *1ST Medifast Meal*	Medifast Plus for Diabetics Vanilla Shake stirred into 1 cup of coffee
MID-MORNING *2ND Medifast Meal*	Medifast Blueberry Oatmeal
LUNCH *Lean & Green Meal*	• 6 oz grilled chicken • 2 cups salad greens with ½ cup mix of diced tomatoes, cucumbers, and green peppers, and 2 Tbsp low-carbohydrate salad dressing
MID-AFTERNOON *3RD Medifast Meal*	Medifast Peanut Butter Crunch Bar
DINNER *Lean & Green Meal*	• 7 oz broiled salmon • Drizzle with mixture of 2 tsp olive oil**, ½ Tbsp lemon juice*, and a dash of dill* • ½ cup wax beans and 1 cup steamed cauliflower with a dash of rosemary*
EVENING *4TH Medifast Meal*	Medifast Chocolate Pudding made with 1 cup skim milk *(healthy snack serving allowed on this specialized plan)*

*optional condiment **healthy fat serving

5 & 2 & 2 Meal Plan

If you have diabetes, your physician may recommend a meal plan that is higher in calories. Here is a sample of our 5 & 2 & 2 Plan, which you can learn more about in the Medifast for Diabetes Guide. This meal plan includes 5 Medifast Meals, 2 Lean & Green Meals, and 2 Healthy Snacks. Talk to your doctor about which meal plan is right for you. All meal plans should include at least **eight** 8-ounce glasses of water (64 ounces total) each day.

Meal Plan for People with Diabetes

(taken from the Medifast for Diabetes Guide)

BREAKFAST *1ST Medifast Meal*	Medifast Blueberry Oatmeal • 8 oz low-fat, sugar-free yogurt**
MID-MORNING *2ND Medifast Meal*	Medifast Hot Cocoa
LUNCH *3RD Medifast Meal and 1ST Lean & Green Meal*	Medifast Banana Pudding • 5 oz grilled salmon • 2 cups salad greens with ½ cup mix of diced cucumbers, peppers, radishes, and celery, and 2 Tbsp low-carbohydrate salad dressing*
MID-AFTERNOON *4TH Medifast Meal*	Medifast Plus for Diabetics Vanilla Shake
DINNER *2ND Lean & Green Meal*	• 6 oz turkey (white meat) • ½ cup brown rice** • 1-½ cups mixed wax and green beans
EVENING *5TH Medifast Meal*	Medifast Plus for Diabetics Strawberry Shake

*optional condiment **healthy snack serving allowed on this specialized plan

Sample Maintenance Meal Plans

Meal Plan 1 (approximately 1,500 calories)

BREAKFAST	Medifast Scrambled Eggs
MID-MORNING	Medifast Maple & Brown Sugar Oatmeal mixed with 1 cup blueberries
LUNCH	• ½ deli sandwich: 3 oz roast beef, 1 slice rye bread, lettuce, tomato, and onion, 1 Tbsp mustard, 1 tsp mayonnaise
MID-AFTERNOON	• 1 cup low-fat yogurt
DINNER	• 5 oz baked tilapia fillet • 1 cup cooked spinach and 2 cups salad greens with ½ cup mix of diced carrots, radishes, cucumbers, tomatoes, and green peppers, and 1-2 Tbsp reduced-fat salad dressing • 1 cup fat-free milk
EVENING	Medifast Oatmeal Raisin Crunch Bar

Meal Plan 2 (approximately 1,500 calories)

BREAKFAST	• ¾ cup high-fiber cereal (>5g of fiber per serving) with ½ cup strawberries and 1 cup skim milk
MID-MORNING	Medifast Cappuccino
LUNCH	• 1 cup low-fat cottage cheese • ½ cup canned pineapple packed in juice • 2 cups salad greens with 2 Tbsp reduced-fat salad dressing*
MID-AFTERNOON	Medifast Cream of Tomato Soup sprinkled with parsley
DINNER	• 4 oz baked chicken breast • 1 cup asparagus topped with 1 tsp margarine
EVENING	Medifast Peanut Butter Crunch Bar • ½-1 cup low-fat yogurt

*vegetable portion divided between lunch and dinner meals

Sample Transition Meal Plans

Stage 1

Week 1	5 Medifast Meals, 1 Lean & Green Meal, and an additional cup of any vegetables.
BREAKFAST	Medifast Cappuccino
MID-MORNING	Medifast Apple Cinnamon Oatmeal with ½ tsp cinnamon
LUNCH	Medifast Chicken & Wild Rice Soup • 2 cups salad greens with ½ cup mix of diced cucumbers, tomatoes, and green peppers, and 1-2 Tbsp reduced-calorie salad dressing
MID-AFTERNOON	Medifast Tropical Punch Fruit Drink
DINNER	• 5 oz lean beef • 1 cup grilled portabella mushrooms
EVENING	Medifast Oatmeal Raisin Crunch Bar

Stage 2

Week 2	4 Medifast Meals, 1 Lean & Green Meal, an additional cup of any vegetables, and a serving of fruit.
BREAKFAST	Medifast Blueberry Oatmeal
MID-MORNING	Medifast Dutch Chocolate 55 Shake with 1-2 tsp sugar-free cherry syrup
LUNCH	Medifast Homestyle Chili • 2 cups salad greens with ½ cup mix of diced cucumbers, tomatoes, and green peppers, and 1-2 Tbsp reduced-calorie salad dressing
MID-AFTERNOON	• 1 cup cantaloupe cubes
DINNER	• 5 oz grilled tuna • 1 cup cooked asparagus drizzled with 1 tsp olive oil and lemon juice*
EVENING	Medifast Peanut Butter Crunch Bar

*optional condiment

Sample Transition Meal Plans

Stage 3

Week 3	4 Medifast Meals, 1 Lean & Green Meal, an additional cup of any vegetables, a serving of fruit, and a serving of dairy.
BREAKFAST	Medifast Hot Cocoa
MID-MORNING	Medifast Peach Flavored Oatmeal
LUNCH	• 6 oz skinless turkey (white meat) • 1 cup broccoli
MID-AFTERNOON	Medifast Vanilla Pudding mixed with ½ cup strawberries
DINNER	Medifast Cream of Chicken Soup • 2 cups salad greens with ½ cup mix of diced cucumbers, tomatoes, and green peppers, and 1-2 Tbsp reduced-calorie salad dressing
EVENING	• ½ cup low-fat, sugar-free yogurt

Stage 4

Weeks 4-12	3 Medifast Meals, 1 Lean & Green Meal, an additional cup of any vegetables, 2 servings of fruit, 2 servings of dairy, an additional 4-6 oz of lean meat, and 1 serving of whole grain.
BREAKFAST	• ¾ cup high-fiber breakfast cereal (>5g of fiber per serving) with 1 cup berries and 1 cup skim milk
MID-MORNING	Medifast Chai Latte
LUNCH	• 4 oz roasted turkey over 2 cups salad greens with ½ cup mix of diced cucumbers, tomatoes, and green peppers, and 1-2 Tbsp reduced-fat salad dressing
MID-AFTERNOON	Medifast Cream of Chicken Soup
DINNER	• 5 oz poached salmon • 1 small baked sweet potato
EVENING	Medifast Banana Pudding made with 1 cup milk and 1 small banana, sliced

References

1. Vasan RS, Pencina MJ, Cobain M, Freiberg MS, D'Agostino RB. "Estimated Risks for Developing Obesity in the Framingham Heart Study." *Annals of Internal Medicine.* 2005; 143:473-480.

2. Bray GA, Nielsen SJ, Popkin BM. "Consumption of high-fructose corn syrup in beverages may play a role in the epidemic of obesity." *American Journal of Clinical Nutrition.* 2004; 79(4):537-543.

3. Critser, G. *Fat Land.* 2003. First Mariner Books, NY NY.

4. Hannum SM, Carson L, Evans EM, *et al.* "Use of portion-controlled entrees enhances weight loss in women." *Obesity.* 2004; 12(3):538-546.

5. Raynor HA, Jeffery RW, Phelan S, Hill JO, Wing RR. "Amount of food group variety consumed in the diet and long-term weight loss maintenance." *Obesity.* 2005;13:883-890.

6. Comings DE, Blum K. "Reward deficiency syndrome: genetic aspects of behavioral disorders." *Progress in Brain Research.* 2000; 126:325-341.

7. Epstein LH, Truesdale R, Wojcik A, Paluch RA, Raynor HA. "Effects of deprivation on hedonics and reinforcing value of food." *Physiology & Behavior.* 2003; 78:221-227.

8. Bardo MT. "Neuropharmacological mechanisms of drug reward: Beyond dopamine in the nucleus accumbens." *Critical Reviews in Neurobiology.* 1998; 12:37-67.

9. Bechara A, Harrington F, Nader K, van der Kooy D. "Neurobiology of motivation: double dissociation of two motivational mechanisms mediating opioid reward in drug-naive versus drug-dependent animals." *The Journal of Neuroscience.* 1992; 106:798-907.

10. Bechara A, Nader K, van der Kooy D. "A two-separate-motivational-systems hypothesis of opioid addiction." *Pharmacology, Biochemistry, & Behavior.* 1998; 59:1-17.

11. Blackburn JR, Phillips AG, Jakubovic A, Fibiger HC. "Dopamine and preparatory behavior: A neurochemical analysis." *Behavioral Neuroscience.* 1989; 103:15-23.

12. Mela DJ. "Determinants of food choice: relationships with obesity and weight control." *Obesity Research*. 2001; 9(4):249S-255S.

13. Noble EP, Blum K, Ritchie T, Montgomery A, Sheridan PJ. "Allelic association of the D2 dopamine receptor gene with receptor-binding characteristics in alcoholism." *Archives of General Psychiatry*. 1991; 48(7):648-654.

14. Volkow ND, Fowler JS. "Addiction, a disease of compulsion and drive: involvement of the orbitofrontal cortex." *Cerebral Cortex*. 2000; 10: 318-325.

15. Hietala J, West C, Syvalahti E, *et al.* "Striatal D2 dopamine receptor binding characteristics in vivo in patients with alcohol dependence." *Psychopharmacology*. 1994; 116(3):285-290.

16. Wang H, Moriwaki A, Wang JB, Uhl GR, Pickel VM. "Ultrastructural immunocytochemical localization of mu-opioid receptors in dendritic targets of dopaminergic terminals in the rat caudate-putamen nucleus." *Neuroscience*. 1997; 81(3):757-771.

17. Blum K, Sheridan L, Wood RC, Braverman ER, Chon JH, Gull JG, Comings DE. "The D2 dopamine receptor gene as determinant of reward deficiency syndrome." *Journal of the Royal Society of Medicine*. 1996; 89:396-400.

18. Noble EP, Noble RE, Ritchie T, *et al.* "D2 dopamine receptor gene and obesity." *International Journal of Eating Disorders*. 1994; 15(3):205-217.

19. Pohjalainen T, Rinne JO, Nagren K, Lehikoinen P, Anttila K, Syvalahti EK, Hietala J. "The A1 allele of the human D2 dopamine receptor gene predicts low D2 receptor availability in healthy volunteers." *Molecular Psychiatry*. 1998; 3(3):256-260.

20. Thompson J, Thomas N, Singleton A, *et al.* "D2 dopamine receptor gene (DRD2) Taq 1A polymorphism: reduced dopamine D2 receptor binding in the human striatum associated with the A1 allele." *Pharmacogenetics*. 1997; 7(6):479-484.

21. Davis LM, *et al.* "Bromocriptine administration reduces hyperphagia and adiposity and differentially affects dopamine D2 receptor and transporter binding in leptin-receptor-deficient zucker rats and rats with diet-induced obesity." *Neuroendocrinology*. 2008; Nov 4.

22. Wang GJ, Volkow ND, Logan J, *et al.* "Brain dopamine and obesity." *The Lancet*. 2001; 357:345-357.

23. Belluzzi A, Brignola C, *et al.* "Effect of an enteric-coated fish oil preparation on relapses in Crohn's disease." *New England Journal of Medicine.* 1996; 334:1557-1560.

24. Kabir *et al.* "Treatment for 2 months with n-3 polyunsaturated fatty acids reduces adiposity and some atherogenic factors but does not improve insulin sensitivity in women with type 2 diabetes: a randomized controlled study." American Journal of Clinical Nutrition. 2007: 86; 1670-1679.

25. Halliwell B, Gutteridge JMC. "Role of free radicals and catalytic metal ions in human disease: an overview." *Methods of Enzymology.* 1990; 186: 1-85.

26. Shen HM, Shi CY, Shen Y, Ong CN. "Detection of elevated reactive oxygen species level in cultured rat hepatocytes treated with aflatoxin B-1." *Free Radical Biology & Medicine.* 1996; 2:139-146.

27. Cui K, Luo X, Xu K, Ven Murthy MR. "Role of oxidative stress and neurodegeneration: recent developments in assay methods for oxidative stress and nutraceutical antioxidants." *Progress in Neuro-Psychopharmacology and Biological Psychiatry.* 2004; 28:771-799.

28. U.S. Department of Agriculture. Oxygen Radical Absorbance Capacity (ORAC) of selected foods. http:/www.ars.usda.gov/nutrientdata. 2007.

29. Baur JA, Sinclair DA. "Therapeutic potential of resveratrol: the in vivo evidence." *National Review of Drug Discovery.* 2006; 5:493-506.

30. Burggraf F. *The CAMP System: Learning to Live in Balance and Harmony With Food 2000.* DayOne Publishing, Charlotte Hall, MD.

31. Appel LJ, Sacks FM, Carey VJ, *et al.* "Effects of protein, monounsaturated fat, and carbohydrate intake on blood pressure and serum lipids: results of the OmniHeart randomized trial." *Journal of the American Medical Association.* 2005 Nov 16; 294(19):2497-8.

32. Nagata C, Takatsuka N, Shimizu H. "Soy and fish oil intake and mortality in a Japanese community." *American Journal of Epidemiology.* 2002; 156(9):824-831.

33. Lukaczer D, Liska DJ, Lerman RH, Darland G, Schiltz B, Tripp M, Bland JS. "Effect of a low glycemic index diet with soy protein and phytosterols on CVD risk factors in postmenopausal women." *Nutrition.* 2006; 22(2):104-113.

34. Davis J, Steinle J, Higginbotham DA, Oitker J, Peterson RG, Banz WJ. "Soy protein influences insulin sensitivity and cardiovascular risk in male lean SHHF rats." *Hormone and Metabolic Research.* 2005; 37(5):309-315.

35. Azadbakht L, Kimiagar M, Mehrabi Y, Esmaillzadeh A,·Padyab M, Hu FB, Willet WC. "Soy inclusion in the diet improves features of metabolic syndrome: a randomized crossover study in postmenopausal women." *The American Journal of Clinical Nutrition.* 2007; 85(3):735-741.

36. Weir HK, Thun MJ, Hankey BR, *et al.* "Annual report to the nation on the status of cancer, 1975-200, featuring the uses of surveillance data for cancer prevention and control." *Journal of the National Cancer Institute.* 2003; 95:1276-1299.

37. Ji BT, Chow WH, Yang G, *et al.* "Dietary habits and stomach cancer in Shanghai, China." *International Journal of Cancer.* 1998; 76:659-664.

38. Lee JK, Park BJ, Yoo KY, Ahn YO. "Dietary factors and stomach caner: a case-control study in Korea." *International Journal of Epidemiology.* 1995; 24:33-41.

39. Nagata C, Takatsuka N, Kawakami N, Shimizu H. "A prospective cohort study of soy product intake and stomach cancer death." *British Journal of Cancer.* 2002; 7:31-36.

40. You WC, Blot WJ, Chang YS, *et al.* "Diet and high risk of stomach cancer in Shandong, China." *Cancer Research.* 1988; 48:3518-3523.

41. Shinchi K, Ishii H, Imanishi K, Kono S. "Relationship of cigarette smoking, alcohol use, and dietary habits with *Helicobacter pylori* infection in Japanese men." *Scandinavian Journal of Gastroenterology.* 1997; 32: 651-655.

42. Heart Disease and Stroke Statistics 2004 Update. Dallas, Texas: American Heart Association; 2003.

43. Stampfer MJ, Hennekens CH, Manson JE, Colditz GA, Rosner B, Willett WC. "Vitamin E consumption and the risk of coronary disease in women." *New England Journal of Medicine.* 1993; 328:1444-9.

44. Lotufo PA, Chae CU, Ajani UA, Hennekens CH, Manson JE. "Male pattern baldness and coronary heart disease: the Physician's Health Study." *Archives of Internal Medicine.* 2000; 160(13):2064-2065.

45. Teixeira SR, Tappenden KA, Carson L, Jones R, Prabhudesai M, Marshall WP, Erdman JW Jr. "Isolated soy protein consumption reduces urinary albumin excretion and improves the serum lipid profile in men with type 2 diabetes mellitus and nephropathy." *Journal of Nutrition.* 2004; 134(8):1874-1880.

46. Cavin C, Delannoy M, Malnoe A, Debefve E, Touche A, Courtois D, Schilter B. "Inhibition of the expression and activity of cyclo-oxygenase-2 by chicory root extract." *Biochemical and Biophysical Research Communications.* 2005; 327(3):742-749.

47. Arterburn DE, Crane PK, Veenstra DL. "The efficacy and safety of sibutramine for weight loss: a systematic review." *Archives of Internal Medicine.* 2004; 164(9):994-1003.

48. Hollander PA, Elbein SC, Hirsch IB, *et al.* "Role of orlistat in the treatment of obese patients with type 2 diabetes. A 1-year randomized double-blind study." *Diabetes Care.* 1998; 21(8):1288-1294.

49. Davidson MH, Hauptman J, DiGirolamo M, *et al.* "Weight control and risk factor reduction in obese subjects treated for 2 years with orlistat: a randomized controlled trial." *Journal of the American Medical Association.* 1999; 281(3):235-242.

50. Finer N, James WP, Kopelman PG, Lean ME, Williams G. "One-year treatment of obesity: a randomized, double-blind, placebo-controlled, multicentre study of orlistat, a gastrointestinal lipase inhibitor." *International Journal of Obesity and Related Metabolic Disorders.* 2000; 24(3):306-313.

51. Heymsfield SB, Segal KR, Hauptman J, *et al.* "Effects of weight loss with orlistat on glucose tolerance and progression to type 2 diabetes in obese adults." *Archives of Internal Medicine.* 2000; 160(9):1321-1326.

52. Rossner S, Sjostrom L, Noack R, Meinders AE, Noseda G. "Weight loss, weight maintenance, and improved cardiovascular risk factors after 2 years treatment with orlistat for obesity." European Orlistat Obesity Study Group. *Obesity.* 2000; 8(1):49-61.

53. Kelley DE, Bray GA, Pi-Sunyer FX, Klein S, Hill J, Miles J, Hollander P. "Clinical efficacy of orlistat therapy in overweight and obese patients with insulin-treated type 2 diabetes: A 1-year randomized controlled trial." *Diabetes Care.* 2002; 25(6):1033-1041.

54. Miles JM, Leiter L, Hollander P, et al. "Effect of orlistat in overweight and obese patients with type 2 diabetes treated with metformin." *Diabetes Care.* 2002; 25(7):1123-1128.

**The study was also presented at the American Diabetes Association's 65th Annual Scientific Session, 2005.*

55. Torgerson JS, Hauptman J, Boldrin MN, Sjostrom L. "Xenical in the prevention of diabetes in obese subjects (XENDOS) study: a randomized study of orlistat as an adjunct to lifestyle changes for the prevention of type 2 diabetes in obese patients." *Diabetes Care.* 2004; 27(1):155-161.

56. Anderson JW, Greenway FL, Fujioka K, Gadde KM, McKenney J, O'Neil PM. "Buproprion SR enhances weight loss: a 48-week double-blind, placebo-controlled trial." *Obesity.* 2002; 10(7):633-641.

57. Gadde KM, Franciscy DM, Wagner HR II, Krishnan KR. "Zonisamide for weight loss in obese adults: a randomized controlled trial." *Journal of the American Medical Association.* 2003; 289(14):1820-1825.

58. Bray GA, Hollander P, Klein S, Kushner R, Levy B, Fitchet M, Perry BH. "A 6-month randomized, placebo-controlled, dose-ranging trial of topiramate for weight loss in obesity." *Obesity.* 2003; 11(6):722-733.

59. Astrup A, Caterson I, Zelissen P, Guy-Grand B, Carruba M, Levy B, Sun X, Fitchet M. "Topiramate: long-term maintenance of weight loss induced by a low-calorie diet in obese subjects." *Obesity.* 2004; 12(10):1658-69.

60. Wilding J, Van Gaal L, Rissanen A, Vercruysse F, Fitchet M. "A randomized double-blind placebo-controlled study of the long-term efficacy and safety of topiramate in the treatment of obese subjects." *International Journal of Obesity and Related Metabolic Disorders.* 2004 Nov; 28(11):1399-410.

61. Wadden TA, Berkowitz RI, Womble LG, Sarwer DB, Phelan S, Cato

RK, Hesson LA, Osei SY, Kaplan R, Stunkard AJ. "Randomized trial of lifestyle modification and pharmacotherapy for obesity." *New England Journal of Medicine.* 2005; 353(20):2111-20.

62. Shara M, Ohia SE, Yasmin T, *et al.* "Dose- and time-dependent effects of a novel (-)-hydroxycitric acid extract on body weight, hepatic and testicular lipid peroxidation, DNA fragmentation and histopathological data over a period of 90 days." *Molecular and Cellular Biochemistry.* 2003 Dec; 254(1-2):339-346.

63. Lydeking-Olsen E, Beck-Jensen JE, Setchell KD, Holm-Jensen T. "Soymilk or progesterone for prevention of bone loss—a 2 year randomized, placebo-controlled trial." *European Journal of Nutrition.* 2004; 43(4): 246-257.

64. Lund TD, Munson DJ, Haldy ME, Setchell KD, Lephart ED, Handa RJ. "Equol is a novel anti-androgen that inhibits prostate growth and hormone feedback." *Biology of Reproduction.* 2004; 70(4):1188-1195.

65. Bacon CG, Mittleman MA, Kawachi I, Giovannucci E, Glasser DB, Rimm EB. "Sexual function in men older than 50 years of age: results from the health professionals follow-up study." *Annals of Internal Medicine*. 2003; 139:161-168.

66. Van Gaal LF, Rissanen AM, Scheen AJ, Ziegler O, Rossner S. "Effects of the cannabinoid-1 receptor blocker rimonabant on weight reduction and cardiovascular risk factors in overweight patients: 1-year experience from the RIO-Europe study." *Lancet*. 2005; 365(9468):1389-97.

67. Cheskin, LJ, *et al*. "Efficacy of meal replacements versus a standard food-based diet for weight loss in type 2 diabetes." *The Diabetes Educator*. Jan/Feb 2008; 34(1):118-127.*

68. Crowell MD, Cheskin LJ. "Multicenter evaluation of health benefits and weight loss on the Medifast weight management program." The Johns Hopkins University School of Medicine.

69. Volkow ND, Fowler JS. "Addiction, a disease of compulsion and drive: involvement of the orbitofrontal cortex." *Cerebral Cortex*. 2000; 10: 318-325.

70. Fagi AS, Johnson WD, Morrissey RL, McCormick DL. "Reproductive toxicity assessment of chronic dietary exposure to soy isoflavones in male rats." *Hormone and Metabolic Research*. 2005; 37(5):309-315.

71. Alekel DL, Germain AS, Peterson CT, Hanson KB, Stewart JW, Toda T. "Isoflavone-rich soy protein isolate attenuates bone loss in the lumbar spine of perimenopausal women." *The American Journal of Clinical Nutrition*. 2000; 72(3):844-852.

72. Giampietro PG, Bruno G, Furcolo G, Casati A, Brunetti E, Spadoni GL, Galli E. "Soy protein formulas in children: no hormonal effects in long-term feeding." *Journal of Pediatric Endocrinology and Metabolism*. 2004; 17(2):191-196.

73. Jemal A, Thomas A, Murray T, Thun M. "Cancer statistics." *Cancer Journal for Clinicians*. 2002; 52:23-47.

74. Borgman M, McErlean E. "What is the metabolic syndrome? Prediabetes and cardiovascular risk." *Journal of Cardiovascular Nursing*. 2006; 21(4):285-290.

75. Gehm BD, McAndrews JM, Chien PY, Jameson JL. "Resveratrol, a polyphenolic compound found in grapes and wine, is an agonist for the estrogen receptor." *The Proceedings of the National Academy of Sciences Online: USA*. 1997; 94:14138-14143.

76. Arjmandi BH, Lucas EA, Khalil DA, et al. "One year soy protein supplementation has positive effects on bone formation markers but not bone density in postmenopausal women." *Journal of Nutrition*. 2005; 4:8.

77. Ngoan LT, Mizoue T, Fujino Y, Tokui N, Yoshimura T. "Dietary factors and stomach cancer mortality." *British Journal of Cancer*. 2002; 87:37-42.

78. Kostelac D, Rechkemmer G, Briviba K. "Phytoestrogens modulate binding response of estrogen receptors alpha and beta to the estrogen response element." *Journal of Molecular Biology*. 2003; 326:77-92.

79. Mai Z, Blackburn GL, Zhou JR. "Soy phytochemicals synergistically enhance the preventative effect of tamoxifen on the growth of estrogen-dependent human breast carcinoma in mice." *Carcinogenesis*. 2007.

80. Lydeking-Olsen E, Beck-Jensen JE, Setchell KD, Holme-Jensen T. "Soymilk or progesterone for prevention of bone loss—a 2 year randomized, placebo-controlled trial." *European Journal of Nutrition*. 2004; 43(4):246-257.

81. Ziegler RG, Hoover RN, Pike MC, et al. "Migration patterns and breast cancer risk in Asian-American women." *Journal of National Cancer Institute*. 1993; 85:1819-1827.

82. Reinwald S, Weaver CM. "Soy isoflavones and bone health: A double-edged sword?" *Journal of Natural Products*. 2006; 69:450-459.

83. Witte JS, Longnecker MP, Bird CL, Lee ER, Frankl HD, Haile RW. "Relation of vegetable, fruit, and grain consumption to colorectal adenomatous polyps." *American Journal of Epidemiology*. 1996; 144: 1015-1025.

84. Yan L, Spitznagel EL. "Meta-analysis of soy food and risk of prostate cancer in men." *International Journal of Cancer*. 2005; 117(4):667-669.

85. Setchell KD, Lydeking-Olsen E. "Dietary phytoestrogens and their effect on bone: evidence from in vitro and in vivo, human observational, and dietary intervention studies." *The American Journal of Clinical Nutrition*. 2003; 78(3):593S-609S.

86. Bennink MR. "Dietary soy reduces colon carcinogenesis in human and rats." *Advances in Experimental Medicine and Biology*. 2001; 492:11-17.

87. Fukuda M, Miyamoto K, Hashizume R, *et al.* "Breast Cancer." *Gan To Kagaku Ryoho*. 2002; 29:1900-1906.

88. Clair RS, Anthony M. "Soy, isoflavones and atherosclerosis." *Handbook of Experimental Pharmacology*. 2005; 170:301-323.

89. Jayagopal V, Albertzaai P, Kilpatrick ES, *et al.* "Beneficial effects of soy phytoestrogen intake in postmenopausal women with type 2 diabetes." *Diabetes Care*. 2002; 25:1709.

90. Casini ML, Marelli G, Papaleo E, Ferrari A, D'Ambrosio F, Unfer V. "Psychological assessment of the effects of treatment with phytoestrogens on postmenopausal women: a randomized, double-blind, crossover, placebo-controlled study." *Fertility and Sterility*. 2006; 85(4):972-978.

91. Hoshiyama Y, Sekine T, Sasaba T. "A case-control study of colorectal cancer and its relation to diet, cigarettes, and alcohol consumption in Saitama Prefecture, Japan." *Tohoku Journal of Experimental Medicine*. 1993; 171:153-165.

92. Geller SE, Studee L. "Soy and red clover for mid-life and aging." *Climacteric*. 2006; 9(4):245-263.

93. Horiuchi T, Onouchi T, Takahashi M, Ito H, Orimo H. "Effect of soy protein on bone metabolism in postmenopausal Japanese women." *Osteoporosis International*. 2000; 11(8): 721-724.

94. Cardoso JR, Baso SN. "Effects of chronic exposure to soy meal containing diet or soy derived isoflavones supplement on semen production and reproductive system of male rabbits." *Animal Reproductive Science*. 2007; 97(3-4):237-245.

95. Health and Welfare Statistics Association. "Life table." (In Japanese). *Journal of Health and Welfare Statistics*. 1999; 46:73.

96. Nishi M, Yoshida K, Hirata K, Miyake H. "Eating habits and colorectal cancer." *Oncology Report*. 1997; 4:995-998.

97. Merritt RJ, Jenks BH. "Safety of soy-based infant formulas containing isoflavones: the clinical evidence." *Journal of Nutrition*. 2004; 134(5):1220S-1224S.

98. Lund TD, Munson DJ, Haldy ME, Setchell KDR, Lephart ED, Handa, RJ. "Equol is a novel anti-androgen that inhibits prostate growth and hormone feedback." *Biology of Reproduction*. 2004; 70:1188-1195.

99. Messina M, Redmond G. "Effects of soy protein and soybean isoflavones on thyroid function in healthy adults and hypothyroid patients: a review of the relevant literature." *Thyroid*. 2006; 16(3):249-258.

100. Peterson G, Barnes S. "Genistein inhibits both estrogen and growth factor-stimulated proliferation of human breast cancer cells." *Cell Growth and Proliferation*. 1996; 7:1345-1351.

101. Morabito N, Crisafulli A, Vergara C, *et al.* "Effects of genistein and hormone-replacement therapy on bone loss in early postmenopausal women: a randomized double-blind placebo-controlled study." *Journal of Bone and Mineral Research*. 2002; 17(10):1904-1912.

102. Trock BJ, Hilakivi-Clarke R. "Meta-Analysis of Soy Intake and Breast Cancer Risk." *Journal of National Cancer Research*. 2006; 98(7):459-471.

103. Halliwell B. "Reactive oxygen species in living systems." *American Journal of Medicine*. 1991; 91:14S-22S.

104. Halliwell B, Gutteridge JMC. "Role of free radicals and catalytic metal ions in human disease: an overview." *Methods of Enzymology*. 1990; 186: 1-85.

105. Rowe B, Davis L. *Anti-inflammatory Foods for Health*. Massachusetts: Fair Winds Press, 2008.

106. Morvarid K, Skurnik G, Naour N, Pechtner V, *et al.* "Treatment for 2 months with n-3 polyunsaturated fatty acids reduces adiposity and some atherogenic factors but does not improve insulin sensitivity in women with type 2 diabetes: a randomized controlled study." *The American Journal of Clinical Nutrition*. 2007; 86:1670-1679.

Index

American Diabetes Association 17, 144, 145, 203
American Obesity Association (AOA) 126, 144, 153, 156
Amino acids 23, 122, 126, 142, 152
Antioxidants 41, 43-48, 122, 126, 134, 138, 150-152, 201
Arthritis 35, 36, 110, 141, 143, 153-155, 168
Bad fats 10, 37, 42
Baldness 134, 136-138, 202
Basal Metabolic Rate 80, 84-87, 92, 93
Benign Prostatic Hypertrophy (BPH) 136
Black cohosh 122, 124
Borg Scale 107, 108
Branched chain amino acids 122, 152
Breast cancer 115, 124-127, 206-208
C-reactive protein 36, 37, 43
Canola oil 10, 37, 91 ,182, 187
Carnitine 152
Chaste tree berry 122, 124
Chicory root extract 142, 153, 155, 203
Cholesterol 5, 11, 15-18, 23, 35, 36, 41-43, 52, 72, 91, 110, 114, 118, 126, 129, 134, 135, 137, 139, 140, 143, 146-152, 156, 160, 163, 167, 178-184
Chondroitin 142, 154
Chromium 142, 145
Citrus bioflavonoids 142, 151, 152
Coenzyme Q10 122, 126, 142, 151, 152
Coronary heart disease (CHD) 45, 125, 126, 141, 143, 146, 148, 152, 202
Daidzein 127, 128, 138
Diabetes vii, 5, 16, 17, 35-37, 41, 44, 47, 59, 71, 100, 110, 114, 120, 139, 141, 143-146, 148, 153, 155, 156, 163, 168, 194, 195, 203, 204, 205
Dihydrotesterone 137
Dopamine 12, 26-31, 124, 161, 162, 164, 165, 199, 200
Dumping Syndrome 168, 171

Echinacea 122, 125
Energy balance 101, 166, 167
Erectile dysfunction 134, 138, 139
Exercise 5, 12, 34, 41, 47, 50, 55, 56, 65, 66, 85, 86, 94, 95, 97, 100, 101-111, 112, 130, 132, 139, 160, 173, 193, 201
Fiber 10, 11, 19-21, 23, 31, 32, 74, 81-83, 88, 90, 97, 121, 122, 133, 150, 151, 163, 166, 178-181, 196, 198
Flexibility 97, 103-105, 108, 109
Food and drug administration (FDA) 23, 42, 114, 126, 142, 150, 160, 165
Free radicals 36, 44, 47, 126, 138, 152, 201, 208
Fullness Index™ 31, 32
Gastric bypass 5, 157, 167-172, 174, 176
Genetics 2, 27, 29, 30, 115, 134,
Genistein 127, 128, 134, 137, 151, 207
Glucosamine 154
Glucose 17, 143-145, 203
Glycemic Index (GI) 31, 42, 142, 144, 145, 202
Glycogen 72
Heart muscle 147, 151
High-density lipoprotein (HDL) 42, 114, 126, 134, 148, 149, 150,
High fructose corn syrup (HFCS) 3, 20, 22, 23
Homocysteine 114, 152
Hot flashes 116, 123-125
Inflammation 35-38, 41-44, 48, 114, 125, 127, 152, 154, 155
Insulin 10, 43, 47, 114, 115, 143-146, 163, 201-203, 208
Isoflavones 114-117, 124, 126-128, 134, 137, 151, 205-207
Ketones 72
Lactose intolerance 168, 172
Lean & Green Meal 6, 72, 73, 75, 77, 81-83, 102, 145, 177, 178, 182, 185-195
Lean muscle mass 72, 101, 103, 113, 124, 134
Low-density lipoprotein (LDL) 42, 43, 72, 114, 126, 134, 150, 151, 163
Lycopene 138
Macronutrient 8, 9, 20, 21, 31, 72
Maintenance 5, 16, 18, 32, 34, 43, 46, 47, 77, 79, 83-85, 87, 92, 95-98, 101, 102, 104, 172, 196, 199, 203, 204

Medifast Meals vii, 5, 16-20, 22, 23, 31, 32, 49, 72-77, 81-83, 85, 92, 93, 102, 113, 114, 116, 117, 121, 124, 133, 141, 142, 145, 157, 170-173, 177, 185-195, 197, 198

Menopause 115, 116, 122-127, 134, 142

Mitochondrial burnout 44

Monitor 19, 52, 55, 60, 84, 94, 96, 97, 106, 116, 132, 144, 145, 162, 163

Monounsaturated fats (MUFAs) 10, 41, 43, 91, 92

Multivitamin 164, 170, 172

Muscle 51, 54, 72, 73, 96, 101, 103-105, 108, 123, 143, 147, 151, 152, 161, 162, 164, 165

Norepinephrine 161, 162, 164, 165

Nutrient 8, 11, 20, 23, 37, 40, 47, 72, 75, 103, 104, 114, 116, 138, 146, 150, 151, 168, 169, 172, 201

Obesity vii, 1-5, 7, 8, 14, 22, 26, 27, 30, 35, 59, 100, 133, 138, 146, 147, 156, 159-162, 167, 168, 173, 199, 200, 203, 204

Olive oil 22, 37, 41, 42, 92, 178, 179, 181, 185, 188, 190, 192, 194, 197

Omega-3 fatty acids 10, 23, 89, 38, 39, 40, 48

Omega-6 fatty acids 38, 39, 42

Osteoarthritis 153, 168

Osteoporosis 110, 124, 125, 127, 128, 142, 169, 207

Oxidative stress 35, 36, 43, 44, 47, 48, 201

Oxygen radical absorbance capacity (ORAC) 45-47, 201

Partially hydrogenated oils 10

Perfectionism 62-64

Peri-menopause 122, 123

Physical activity level (PAL) 84-87, 92, 93, 156

Polyunsaturated fats (PUFAs) 10, 37-39, 42, 91, 92, 201, 208

Portion vi, 3, 4, 7, 8, 11, 15-19, 22, 31, 34, 68, 84, 94-97, 99, 102, 103, 108, 144, 145, 158, 171, 172, 189, 193, 196, 199

Prostate cancer 41, 115, 117, 134-138, 206

Pycnogenol 122, 126, 142, 151, 152

Rate of perceived exertion (RPE) 107

Resveratrol 47, 48, 201, 205

Reward Deficiency Syndrome 26, 27, 199, 200

Satiety 19-22, 31, 32

Saturated fat 10, 11, 23, 42, 48, 92, 113, 121, 122, 133, 150

Selenium 138

Serotonin 161, 162, 165

Soy 20, 23, 89, 113-117, 124, 126-128, 134-139, 144, 150, 151, 155, 183, 201, 202, 204-208

Soy protein 19, 20, 23, 113-117, 121, 122, 124, 126-128, 133, 134, 137, 138, 142, 145, 150, 155, 173, 202, 203, 205, 207

Soybeans 37, 89, 92, 113, 114, 128, 138, 150, 151, 207

Stress 3, 4, 11, 34, 44, 56, 94, 95, 97, 103, 111, 115, 148

Super Citrimax 121-123, 133

Super Omega-3 40, 41

Support vii, 4, 5, 10, 33, 41, 45, 50, 57, 61, 71, 74, 96, 97, 114, 120, 131, 132, 140, 141, 174, 175

Testosterone 117, 136-139

Thermic effect of food (TEF) 84

Total energy expenditure (TEE) 84-87

Trans fats 10, 11, 42, 48, 92,

Transition 15, 77, 79-83, 87, 95-98, 123, 197, 198

Triglycerides 17, 36, 126, 146, 150, 152, 163

Type 2 diabetes 17, 36, 114, 143-145, 147, 148, 160, 167, 168, 201, 203, 208

Vegetables 6, 10, 11, 18, 20, 21, 37, 42, 43, 45, 73, 79, 80-83, 87, 89, 90, 91-93, 98, 113, 138, 145, 170, 180-182, 189, 196-198, 206

Vitamins 10, 11, 18, 23, 70, 90, 102, 128, 138, 150-152, 155, 161, 163, 164, 168, 170-172

Water 20, 21, 24, 39, 54, 55, 65, 68, 75-77, 89, 96, 112, 113, 163, 170, 179-195

Whey 23, 121, 128, 133

Yo-Yo Diet 11, 13, 15, 64

Zinc 11, 23, 138